# MUSCLEGASM

## A NEW FACE FOR FITNESS

KEITH NULL

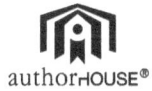
authorHOUSE®

AuthorHouse™ LLC
1663 Liberty Drive
Bloomington, IN 47403
www.authorhouse.com
Phone: 1-800-839-8640

Published by AuthorHouse  03/21/2014

ISBN: 978-1-4918-6219-3 (sc)
ISBN: 978-1-4918-6218-6 (hc)
ISBN: 978-1-4918-6217-9 (e)

Library of Congress Control Number: 2014902385

# CONTENTS

# MUSCLEGASM

Whenever you start any new exercises or diets, always consult with your doctor first. This is very important!!! Some of my exercises can be dangerous to certain populations, so ask your doctor before starting them.

I've have made amazing discoveries in the field of fitness. This book explains theses discoveries.

It's time that I passed on what I know. And what I know is the culmination of experiences that I have observed, and some common sense. I graduated from Temple University with a degree in kinesiology (science of human movement), which is like an auto mechanic for the musculoskeletal system. I also went to a Swedish massage school. My education and real life experiences as a construction worker and athlete, was the perfect blend to understand concepts that nobody has before. I've learned what makes muscles and joints sore and what it takes to "fix" them. I worked with construction workers who had every ach and pain there is. I solved these problems and made same amazing discovers in the process.

This book was created out of necessity. As a construction worker in Philadelphia, I would get the winters off enabling me to obtain a degree in Kinesiology. I didn't work in a large university or hospital. I worked on the roof, where I was able to observe what causes injuries, in real time. I had an advantage over my colleagues that worked in hospitals and health clinics because they only saw clients after the injury has occurred. I was there watching these injuries arising from the beginning. I was able to figure out how to prevent these injuries easily, because I was already on the scene of the injury. I learned to observe people; how someone moves, what their posture is, what kind of work is being performed, what's in their lunchbox, and what are they drinking. Once I discovered a problem with one of these observations, the answer to the problem was usually easy to solve. Believe me, on construction sites you see almost every kind of injury. As a construction worker, an athlete, your health is everything. There are one hundred young guys to take your place if you show any kind of weaknesses. I will relay some of my stories of healing and improving, that I have encountered in my career. The information in this book is what I needed to know to survive on the job. I made many happy coworkers along the way. They say, "necessity is the mother of invention", well; maybe this book is an example of that?

Many problems with our muscles and joints arise from imbalances in the muscles. These problems need to be diagnosed and "fixed". Just like a car would need to be. To "fix" a sore muscle, and or the corresponding joints, it is often one of two things. Either a muscle, or group of muscles, is too weak or they are too strong. When a muscle gets exercised it becomes stronger, it also becomes shorter. Yes the muscle shrinks. This causes imbalances and uneven stress, creating all types of problems. Through my years I have discovered fast and effective ways to make a muscle stronger or weaker, longer or shorter. My weight-training workout "The Whirl" promises that you will get a fast, safe, workout that offers tremendous results in strength and muscle size. My self massage techniques, "The Coach Potato" and "The Ripper", will demonstrate that you can give yourself a deeper, more relaxing massage than any massage therapist can. My stretching exercise called, "Gravity Yoga", will demonstrate how to get the most out of stretching with the aid of gravity. The nutrition segment deals with what is most current and what makes good sense.

Weather old or young, top athlete or in a wheelchair, I guarantee that there is something in this book that can change your life. If you ever had a sore back, this book is for you. Personally, I am 50 years old and I'm stronger and more flexible than I was in High school and I was an all-star athlete. This can happen to you. So hop on board The Musclegasm express. It's going be a fun ride!

Muscles are the most visible things in our bodies that demonstrate our health. They are the indicators of health. When they go bad, then so does our whole body. Muscles make us move and enjoy life. For most of us, muscles are our moneymakers because well condition muscles are vital for work and play.

Most people say they have little time to spend on conditioning their muscles, which are key components of our well-being. Working long hours and family responsibilities makes it difficult to find the time for exercise. However, finding time is a wise investment to your health and happiness. In finical terms, good muscle conditioning increases the ability to generate capital. After all, you can't do your job well if you aren't healthy.

Through my years of experience, education and common sense, I have discovered and streamlined various exercises that will optimize amazing results in a timely manner. I will walk you through a journey of body exploration and discovery. You will learn about yourself and rid yourself of pain,. You will regain the freedom of motion of your youth. In many cases you will become stronger and more flexible that you ever were. If you're a top athlete, then this book will make you even better. If you are an aging or overweight individual, this book will provide information that could be vital.

So why did I title my book, "Musclegasm"? Well, it has to do with the sensation one feels when a chronically stiff muscle or group of muscles suddenly becomes relaxed. It is euphoric and addictive. It is a rush of pleasure. It truly is a muscle orgasm. These musclegasms occur quite frequently when performing my self-massage and stretching techniques. Lets face it; we all have sore muscles at one time, if not all of the time. Some people aren't even aware they have sore muscles until it becomes relaxed and relieved of stress. Often enough, when the muscle becomes relaxed, so does any pain that may be there in a corresponding joint.

This book will demonstrate what it takes to get an athletic, balanced body. My exercises, for the most part, are of my own making. The roots of these exercises are from ancient techniques, modern science and my own inventiveness.

There are no expensive gadgets or machines required for my exercises. These are very low budget exercises. Anyone can afford what is needed and in many cases many of the items are already found in most homes.

Exercise not only is great for the body but it increases your cognitive abilities as well. Yes, it increases your brainpower. Study after study has shown that regular exercise improves memory and even has positive results with people with brain disorders like Alzheimer's disease. Exercise will keep your mind, body and spirit working well into old age.

My experience all started when I was just out of high school visiting my aunt n California. After a day of surfing, I experienced some soreness in my upper back and neck area. This is common amongst surfers, and really everybody. My aunt, who was an Olympic swim coach, showed me a muscle relaxation technique. She basically gave me deep pressure massage with her elbow. My aunt located several tight muscles and proceeded to massage those areas by applying lots of pressure with her elbow. She was applying most of her body weight, pinpointed and focused with her elbow, on my sore muscle. Wow! I was quite surprised at the pain that I was feeling. Just touching those areas was painful, and here was my aunt elbowing me with the whole weight of her body focused on that area. It was almost unbearable, but just as I thought she was crazy, that muscle relaxed. It really was a rush of relaxation. It overwhelmed me. It was my first musclegasm. Just like that, an area of my body that was immobile and in pain, is now free of its misery. I now had movement in my shoulder area that I have never had before. All the pain was gone, It was amazing and I wanted more. Yes! My 82-year-old Aunt gave me my first musclegasm. My aunt (Candice Barton) also demonstrated that something similar can be done by lying on top of a little hard rubber ball. Instead of using an elbow for deep pressure massage, one would simply replace it with the use of a hard rubber ball. This was perfect for my situation, because having my aunt follow me around as my private massage therapist every time I felt pain was not an option. So self-massage was the way to go.

Soon after this experience I graduated for Temple University with a degree in Kinesiology (sports medicine). I quickly then enrolled in a school for Swedish massage. I was now armed with the science and theory that I needed to take my ideas on fitness to the next step. I started work on a self-massage technique that was accomplished by rolling on hard rubber balls in the style of Swedish massage. It provided tremendous results.

I also invented a muscle building technique, with the use of dumbbells, which optimizes training results, while being safe and therapeutic. I call it "The Whirl". The Whirl increases muscle mass faster and safer than many other weight lifting styles that I have seen. In my opinion and what I have seen, the whirl is unmatched in the field of exercise. The Whirl allows you to use less weight with greater results than does conventional weight lifting. The Whirl is safer for you're joints because you use far less weight when performing the Whirl. There is less stress on the joints. Also with conventional weight training, the exercises are performed with the same repetitious movement over and over. This causes the cartilage between the joints to wear unevenly. Kind of like ruts in the road cause by tires repeating going over the same spots. This is not true with The Whirl. Because the Whirl is performed in a circular motion that distributes weight over a greater surface area of the joint cartilage, there isn't any uneven wear. The Whirl is very low impact and safe. Therefore, The Whirl has the potential to be safer than conventional weight lifting and even therapeutic.

The whirl advances weight training to the realm of 3 dimensions. Let me explain. In normal or conventional weight training, all the movements are in a single plane (two dimensional). With the whirl, the body moves are in multiple planes or 3 dimensions. These three dimensional exercises have the benefit of utilizing vastly more muscle fibers and neurons (motor units), than conventional 2 dimensional weight training exercises. These implications for training are huge. If more muscle fibers and neurons are firing, then you receive a better training effect, with regards to muscular strength and size. If more muscle fibers are fatiguing, then more muscle fibers will become stronger, when left to repair. Why just train one group of muscle fibers (as with 2 dimensional exercises), when you can train many, many combinations with my 3 dimensional techniques?

Because of the complex and ever changing movements of The Whirl, these exercises have a resistant to the General Adaptation Syndrome (GAS). General Adaptation Syndrome is a situation where as the body becomes accustomed to a workout routine and is anti-productive for fitness gains. This GAS is a huge obstacle to overcome in weight training, but The Whirl seems to eliminate this problem

To accompany my self-massage and my weight lifting techniques, I have reinvented the art stretching. I call this chapter, "Gravity Yoga". I dedicated it to Bruce Lee, the art of Yoga, and too myself for twisting it all together. Bruce Lee was a man before his time. He refused to conform to the establishment and the conventional ways of the martial arts. He claimed that the martial arts were systematic and predictable. Predictable is not a good thing when it comes to fighting. Lee said the best style of fighting was to have no style. I style which could not be predicted. He was correct. His thinking outside the box is my inspiration.

Gravity Yoga, will describe many stretches that are my own invention and some common stretches. Theses stretches are performed with the utilization and facilitation of gravity. I've discovered how to use gravity in a way that optimizes the stretch. You will get results like never before. I demonstrate how to utilize gravity in a way that forces the body into a correct posture and promotes proper breathing. You may never get a deeper, more relaxing stretch.

My chapter on aerobic fitness explains the importance of this to your health and happiness. I tell you exactly how much you need to get aerobically fit and what are the best techniques. No big inventions here on my part, just science and common sense.

My final chapter on Nutrition, I explain current science and diet recommendations in a simple and easy to understand way. Just because this chapter is last doesn't mean that it is less important. It is now understood that the proper diet can eliminate most, if not all diseases, even cancer. So a good diet is necessary for optimal results with my exercises. A good diet will provide the fuel that is needed to sustain exercise and work. A good diet is what is needed to live long and happy. Without enough protein and other nutrients, building muscle will not happen. Diet and fitness are closely interconnected and you can't have one without the other.

Even if you have no interest, in weight lifting or massage or any of the other chapters, I ask you to please read them anyway. There is information in all the chapters that could be vital and you will learn something. Enjoy the ride.


If you have any questions on any of my topics, online consultation and videos are available at keithnull@comcast.net

# CHAPTER 1

# THE WHIRL

Weight training and particularly dumbbell training has been proven to be one of the most effective ways to build muscle size and strength. Dumbbells are known for there excellent ability to develop core strength and balance. Dumbbells are best for developing large groups of muscle and getting them to work well together in a natural fashion. I take this concept many steps further. I substantially improved on what was already considered the best form of weight training.

The Whirl will can give you greater strength through a wider range of motion than conventional dumbbell training. Granted if you are a power lifter you will want to do the typical weight lifting training, where as you train in a few specific movements for a specific task. For Instance if you are training for competition in the bench press, you will want to train in that specific movement, which is the bench press. But this does not apply to most athletic events or even ordinary life. We do not move in specific movements. We adapt the angles and position of our joints and body parts to corresponds for what is needed at that particular time. Let me explain. As a soccer player, I constantly had to push people off that grabbed me. Every situation was a different set of circumstances that required a slightly different kind of push, requiring slightly different angles of force. Training with a conventional bench press only improves strength in that exact same movement. Slight variations to that movement get little to no improvement in strength. Studies have proven this. Therefore convention weight training does little good when I had to push someone at a slightly different angle or direction than the bench press that I had been training with. Conventional weight training is very restrictive and allows for only small strength gains in a narrow range of motions. A different approach to weight training is needed. One that encompasses greater strength through a wider range of movement is what is needed. Like I said before, The Whirl doesn't limit strength to one particular motion. It provides strength in multiple movements. It requires multiple combinations of muscle fibers contracting to accomplish this whirling movement. Conventional weight training only requires one combination of muscle fibers contracting to create an inline or 2 dimensional movements. My whirl version of the bench press and other exercises, allows for greater strength through a wide range of movements. The whirl works the whole muscle, not just part of muscles, as in conventional weight training exercises. It is more complete!

Not only does The Whirl perform a more complete muscle workout, but it also works more of the stabilizing muscles than does conventional weight training. Stabilizing muscles don't normally move much, but just act to stabilize and control a movement. So now with my whirling bench press, the Latissimus dorsi (lats) and the trapezius (traps) that were once just non-moving stabilizing muscle, are now forced to contract and move, due to the nature of the whirling movements. With The Whirl, not only are the prime moving muscles strengthened better than conventional weight training, but so are the stabilizing muscles. This idea holds true with all my whirling dumbbell exercises. The Whirl is the future so hop on board and get the edge on the competition, and live a longer, more injury free life.

Another problem with weight training in the same repetitious movements can be harmful to your joints. Repetitious movement causes groves and tears to form in the cartilage that lies in your joints betweens the bones. For example, take the conventional bench press again. Many athletes and weight lifters suffer from shoulder injuries because of the same exact bench press movement over and over again. The Whirl eliminates this repetitious wear by the nature of the whirling motion. It's a smooth, circular motion that is buffering to the cartilage. As opposed to the gouging, linear movements of conventional weight training. This whirling motion prevents groves being worn in joint cartilage. Repetitious movements cause inflammation and arthritis. The Whirl is not a repetitious movement. Unlike conventional weight training, the force of The Whirl is spread out over the whole joint cartilage making it safe and even therapeutic. These therapeutic values coupled with the unmatched training effects, makes The Whirl in a class of its own.

As I stated before, The Whirl helps to eliminate General Adaption Syndrome, which creates a plateau of progression in weight training. When the same movements are done over and over again in weight training, the body learns to compensate through other means. In other words, This syndrome halts the progression of the positive effects of your workout. Because The Whirl has such a complex movements that are never really duplicated, and the fact that you are changing direction of the whirl with each set, makes this form of weight training unmatched for counteracting The General Adaption Syndrome.

The Whirl also allows the use of much less weight than conventional dumbbell exercises. In conventional weight training the body moves in a single plane (2 dimensional). Once again, take the conventional bench press. The arms are moving up and downs in a single plan (2 dimensions). The Whirl's motions are in 3 dimensions, with the arms moving up, down and around. This 3 dimensional movement requires many more muscle fibers needed to complete the task. There are possibly a million or more combinations of muscle fibers and neurons that are required with this 3 dimensional whirling movement. When more muscle fibers are being exercised, better muscular growth and strength occurs. The Whirl has great training effects.

This 3-D movement also allows the stabilizer muscles (stabilizers), which normally don't move, to move when weight training. Stabilizers in conventional weight training are under an isometric contraction, which means the muscles stay the same length while contracting. Stabilizers stay in place and assist the movement with conventional weight training. This isometric contraction isn't the best type of muscular contraction for muscle development and strength. Concentric and eccentric contractions are better for muscle development. These types of muscle contractions occur with The Whirl. Concentric and eccentric contraction means that the muscle gets shorter and longer, while under contraction. These muscles are moving and not static. These types of muscle contractions provide a far better training effect than isometric contraction. This is another reason why The Whirl is better than conventional weight training.

The Whirl is a paradox in that it allows for much lighter weights to be lifted, but with a better training effect then conventional weight training. Lighter weights also means less stress on your joints, which means less injuries. The Whirl is outstanding for therapy. The Whirl has healing powers!

There are many ways to increase the resistance when attempting The Whirl. All can be used to customize your workout.

1. Add more weight to the dumbbell
2. Increase the number of whirls
3. Increase the diameter or size of the whirls.
4. Adjust the speed of the whirls.

As you can see there are many variables that will change the resistance for The Whirl. This means there are endless possibilities for different training effects. For instance maybe you want pure strength and size. Well than you might to use heaver weight, with only a few large slow swirls, less reps and more sets. Where as a golfer might want to train with less weight, more swirls, more reps and less sets. The possibilities are endless with The Whirl.

Another hurdle that The Whirl clears that conventional weight training gets tripped on is this. It is had always been a rule with weight training that your last rep of a set should end in complete exhaustion to obtain the best strength results. In other words the last rep of a set ends when you can't do any more. Let's say you are bench-pressing and on the 8th or 9th rep you are exhausted and absolutely can't do one more rep. In fact you were so exhausted that a spotter had to aid you with your last rep. This exactly what you want to do for optimum strength gains… Until now. With The Whirl, you can always perform at least one more rep after complete exhaustion. Unlike conventional weight training, the resistance in The Whirl can be changed by performing less whirls in a rep. It's almost as if removing some weight on the bar, right in the middle of your exercise, which can't be done. Let me explain, lets say you are performing a bench press using my whirl technique. Lets say you hit complete exhaustion on your 8th or 9th rep, but this time you don't have to quit or have a spotter help you. You simple do less whirling action on the next rep. Lets say you were performing 5 whirls for each rep before you reached exhaustion, just perform 3 whirls per rep after you reached exhaustion and what would have other wise been your last rep. The Whirl takes you above and beyond the what was previously considered complete exhaustion. Get with The Whirl. It's going to change everything!

Because the muscles and skeleton operates as levers, situations arise where a particular portion of a lift is easier to perform than other parts. I don't want to get into biomechanics much but this has to do with the force created by contacting muscles (effort), to move a load created by the dumbbell, and the joint acts as the fulcrum. At certain angles or positions there is greater mechanical advantage in the lever system, so the muscle does not have to work as hard to overcome the load. Let me explain, take the bench press, have you ever notice that the beginning of the lift, when the weight is closest to the chest, that the weight is more difficult to lift than at the end of the lift, when the arms are full extended? In this situation, the chest muscles (pectoralis) only have to work hard at the beginning of the lift and don't have to work hard at the end of the lift. This allows the muscle to rest, which is anti-productive when it comes to weight training. This uneven muscle contraction will not produce the same beneficial training results that a continuous contraction will. To correct this problem you must increase the load at the end of the bench press, when arms are fully extended, but this is impossible to do with ordinary dumbbell exercises. However, you may adjust the resistance by changing the speed and size of the whirling motion. This will provide the addition load at the end of a lift. The whirl provides balance muscle contraction throughout the entire lift, yielding increased training results.

Reversing the direction of the whirl each set, will greatly increase the training effects. For example, when attempting the whirling bench press, first set you whirl your right arm in a clockwise and left arm counterclockwise direction. Your hands meet in the center. The second set, you reverse the whirl and rotate your right arm in a counter clockwise direction while the left arm goes clockwise. In other words, each set gets the opposite direction to the whirling motion that was done in the previous set. Once again, these complex movements are beneficial in so many ways.

The Whirl requires a lot of thinking. There is a lot going on mentally. Conventional dumbbell training is considered difficulty because of the focus on balance and form. With The Whirl, there is the added variable of the whirling motion, plus balance and form, and that equals a lot on concentration needed to perform The Whirl. This concentration is a good thing, because the more the mind works, the better the training results. It is a fact that a large part of muscular strength is a result of improved brain and neural function, and not an increase of muscle mass. What happens is when you want to move, the brain sends electrochemical impulses to nerves, called motor neurons. These neurons pass these impulses on to the muscle fibers, causing the muscle fibers to contract and crate a movement. As a muscle gets stronger from training, these impulses occur more rapidly and with improved synchronization and rhythm. This improve cadence in impulses is what's responsible for most of the strength gains, and not an increased muscle mass. Yes, big muscles aren't always as strong as smaller muscles that have better nerve transmission. I always found that interesting. Brainpower!

When I explain to clients that most of muscular strength is derived from the nervous system functioning more efficiently they refuse to believe me. They tell me, "That's not true. I can see my muscles getting bigger after each workout". This is true, your muscles do get bigger, but' the increase in muscle size is do to water. After exercise, the muscles become hydrophilic, which means they swell from water retention, up to 40% water retention. And this water retention is the reason weight lifting programs tend to make people gain weight. The fact is, in most cases there is only a 3% protein gain in muscle mass over a whole year of weight training, the rest is water. All increases in muscle size for a woman is attributed to water gain, and not from adding protein, because women cannot add protein to muscles like men can. However women get the some wonderful benefits that weight training provides. And almost all the strength gains are from neural development. Women can never gain muscle mass from weight training, but they do become toned.

Another thing I always found interesting is, no matter much you lift weights, you can never increase the number of muscle cells. You're born with the number of muscles cells and it never increases. Weight training only increases a muscle cell's diameter. Cats are the only mammals capable of hyperplasia (increase in the number of muscle cells). That's not true with fat cells. One can increase the number and size of fat cells by over eating. Another thing is that you can never eliminate the number of fat cells in your body. You can only make fat cells smaller. You can increase the number of fat cells, and once that happens you can never get rid of them without surgery. Seems a little unfair that you can increase fat cell numbers, but you can't increase the number of muscle cells. Nature's cruel joke.

A 22-year-old male came to me wanted to gain strength. He was a carpenter who did allot lifting drywall and he wanted to train for it, just like an athlete would. He told me that he had been lifting weight for a few years now and had seen little improvement. I directed him to The Whirl and he was impressed. He seen better results with The Whirl in two months then he had with the years of conventional weight training. He told me that he has many his co-workers over his house performing The Whirl.

I like this and all my exercises; I can testify that they work because I practice what I preach.

Dumbbells will be needed to perform The Whirl. I suggest the kind of dumbbells that allows you to adjust the weight. Complete dumbbell set can be expensive but are more convenient. You don't need much weight. As you can see in my photos I'm using 15 lbs or less in each hand for most of my exercises. In addition, some of my exercises are performed with the use of a bench. They can be performed on the floor but are far less effective because it restricts movement. I suggest you get 2 buckets and a blank or wood 4 or 5 ft long by18 inches or so across. Just place the plank on the buckets with a towel over it and you have a cheap bench. Or you can gat a real weight lifting bench, if you have the space and money for one. I try to make these exercises affordable to everyone. I also suggest getting a mirror because form is everything. The mirror is your personal trainer, in that it tells you when your posture is bad, or if one arm is lower that the other, and so on. The mirror lets you know when you are cheating. Cheating is adding movement that aids in your lift. An example would be moving your body forward and backward while performing an arm curl. No cheating! It is important that you keep your back strait. I cannot stress the use of the mirror enough. Place one on the ceiling so you can see yourself on the bench doing fly's and bench presses. Even if you can only afford a cheap mirror that you can move around to accommodate different exercises… Get one!

Here is what I suggest as the most simple, basic, whirling weight workout. It covers all the basics in a timely manor. These 5 simple exercises will give you a well-balanced workout. However feel free to improvise and use your imagination. The whirl can be applied to many types of weight training techniques, even those involving weight machines that use pulleys and cables/

The workout consists of 2 sets, which is less than the conventional dumbbell or barbell workout consisting of 3 or more sets. You don't need that many sets with The Whirl because it is more a complete workout. If you are week in a particular area, than more sets may be desirable. Each set will take about approximately 20 minutes to complete. With 2 sets, total workout will last 40 minutes. Each set will be performed with opposite direction in the whirls. This should be performed at least twice a week but 3 days is best.

Here is my quick list of whirling dumbbell exercises.

1. Whirling Fly's (Done on the bench or floor)
2. Whriling Overhead Press
3. Whirling Arm Curls
4. Whirling Bench press (Push-ups work as well)
5. Whirling Modified Back Fly's

These exercises are a suggestion of well-balanced workout that will take the least amount of time and still yield big results. There are many dumbbell exercises that you can apply The Whirl to. For instance, if you would like to develop your latissimus dorsi "LATS" you can perform some rows with the whirl. What I'm trying to say is that be inventive and customize your workout for your specific strengths and weaknesses.

For the legs I do not recommend The Whirl. The hip girdle does not work mechanically the same as the shoulder girdle. It does not have the same flexibility and movement that the shoulders possess. Plus it's hard to grab dumbbells with your feet. So I do not advise it. However the use of an elliptical machine is a great way to develop your legs. It is a low impact and therapeutic much like The Whirl is. And by the way, an elliptical supplies aerobic exercise, which is vital to health. Aerobic fitness will be discussed in another chapter. The elliptical machine will increase strength. If one desires more strength in the legs, then leg extensions and leg curls are great. Leg extensions and curls are often used as therapy for ailing knees. I do not recommend performing squats for the potential knee damage.

I suggest that you read my nutritional section of this book. Weight training demands that you consume adequate amounts of nutrition for it to be effective. There is much to know about particularly protein requirements. You don't want to take to much or two little. You may want to consider taking a plant based protein supplement. Meat and particularly red meat have many side effects, like associations with cancer.

The Whirl workout is a more complete workout than traditional workout and yields big results. Steroids should be avoided for your long-term health risk. You don't need steroids to get big results with The Whirl. Steroids increase the metabolism, which decreases your age of death.

You also want to be well hydrated whenever you are weight training. You need to flush out toxins like lactic acid from your muscles cells. Lactic acid build up will hinder muscle development and can even kill you in extreme cases. Water also lubricates the joints, brings nutrient's to the cells, aids in digestion, reduces fatigue and increase athletic performance Drink your water!

You should always stretch before strength training like with the Whirl. If you strengthen a stiff muscle, you only make it stiffer, which can lead to additional problems. I suggest the stretches from the chapter "Gravity Yoga", or at least the complimentary stretches at the end of the chapter. Always ask your doctor before starting an exercise program or massage. Stretching after The Whirl will help to rid the body of lactic acid and keep the muscles loose.

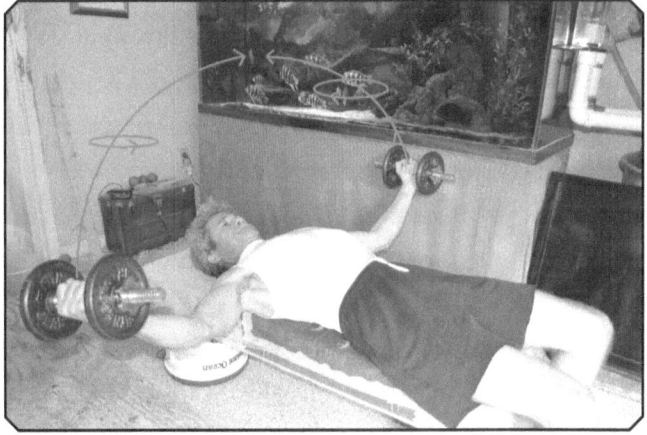

## 1. Whirling Fly

The Whirling Fly thoroughly works the chest area. Where as the conventional fly only works the middle section of the pectoral muscle, The Whirl Fly works the upper, middle and lower sections of the pectoral and more of the deltoid muscle. In addition The Whirl Fly also forces the stabilizer muscles like the trapezius, deltoid, and latissimus dorsi to move and contract concentrically and eccentrically. The biceps also gets worked as a stabilizer. This doesn't happen with the convention dumbbell fly. You are receiving a much more complete workout with The Whirl.

A. Lying on your back, on the bench, grab each dumbbell with each hand and hold at your body height. I prefer the underhand grip but the overhand or any variation of the two will work just fine.

B. Raise the dumbbells with a whirling motion slowly till they are side by side over you. Then lower the dumbbells using the same whirling action. I prefer my whirl size to be about 4 to 12 inches in diameter and like to perform 4 or 5 whirls up and another 4 or 5 whirls down. More whirls can be applied. The whirling motion occurs at the shoulder joint, not the elbow or wrist. The forearms should remain parallel to each other. The right arm performs clockwise whirls and left arm counterclockwise whirls and meet in the center. When attempting the next set, the whirl direction is reversed. Perform 6 to 12 reps. With 2 sets. Never complete sets back to back. Move on to the next exercise when complete.

C. Try to keep the same elbow angle throughout the lift.

D. Breathing out as you raise your arms and breath in when lowering them is what conventional weight training suggested. However I feel you shouldn't get to caught up in the breathing because The Whirl is a slower exercise than conventional dumbbell and your breathing doesn't always synchronize up. Breathing normal is most important. Don't hold your breath. I have seen people pass out from that.

------------------------------------------------------------

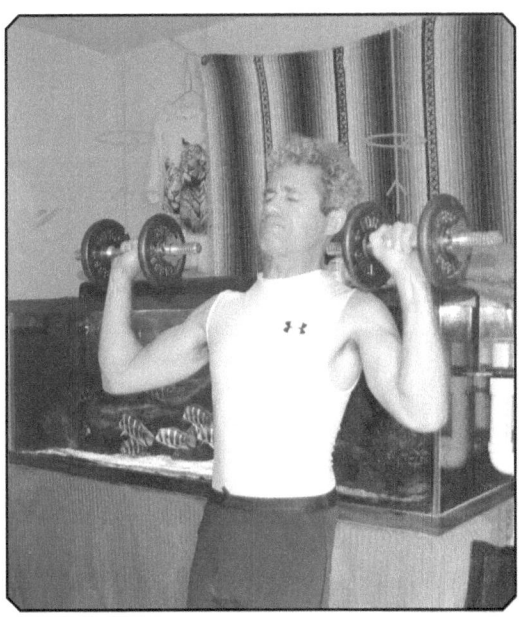

## 2. Whirling Overhead Press

The Whirling Overhand Press develops the mainly the triceps and deltoids muscles. The trapezius, serratus anterior, rotator cuff, latissimus dorsi and rhomboid muscles also get worked better to the whirling motion. The Whirling Overhead Press develops many more muscle combinations than does the conventional overhead press. You will gain strength through a wider range of motion than you do with normal, conventional weight training.

A. Stand or sit on the bench making sure back is strait.
B. Hold the dumbbells at the shoulder with the overhand or underhand grip.
C. Raise the weight slowly, whirling at your arms with 4-12 inches in diameter circles. 4 or five times up and the same 4 or 5 times down. More can be done. The whirling motion occurs at the shoulder joint. The fore arms should remain parallel to each to each other and perpendicular to the floor. Right arm whirls

clockwise and left arm counterclockwise. 6 to 12 reps. Reverse the whirl on the second set.

D.  Breathing normally

---

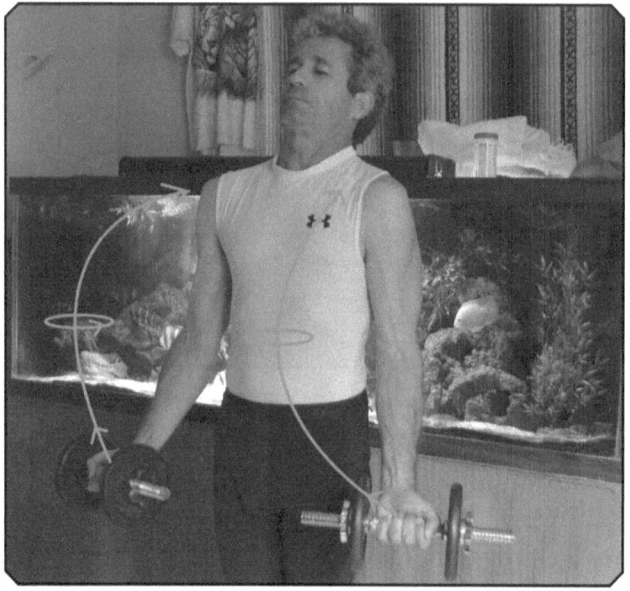

## 3. Whirling Curl

The whirling Curl develops primarily the bicep muscle and the brachioradialis muscle located in the fore arm. The deltoid, muscle also get worked. The Whirling curl works the bicep like no other curl comes close to. You will be able to use far less weight than with the conventional curl, but with better strength results. To me this is one of the most strenuous exercises. It seems that holding the correct form by not swaying the back and cheating, takes considerable energy.

A.  Stand and hold each dumbbell in each hand down the side of the body, palms facing out in the underhand grip.

B. Raise both dumbbells with a swirling motion. The upper arm should not move from position down your side. There is a slight rotation of the upper arm created by the whirl, but the upper arm does not move from position along and down your side. All the movement is done at the elbow. This is different than the overhead press and the fly, where the whirl occurs at the shoulder. 4 or 5 whirls up and 4 or 5 whirls down. 4-12 inch whirls. Right arm clock wise whirl and left counterclockwise for first set and reverse the whirl on the second set.

C. Don't cheat and move your body much. Make sure back and neck are strait.

D. Breath normal

---

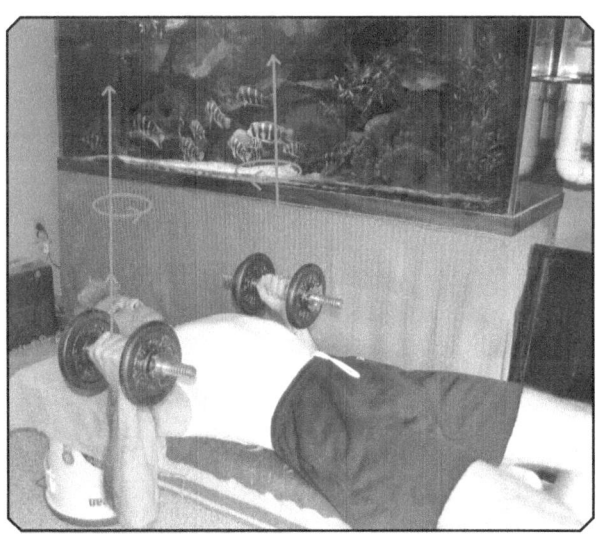

## 4. Whirling Bench Press

The Whirl Bench Press mainly develops the chest muscles that are the upper, middle and lower portions of the pectoralis muscles.

The whirling motion also works the deltoid, triceps, rotator cuff of the shoulder, the rhomboids of the upper back and latissimus dorsi.

1. Lie on your back on the bench and hold the two dumbbells ate chest level along your body with the palms facing each other
2. Raise the dumbbells strait up with about 6 whirls (4-12inches) till the elbows are almost locked. Then lower the arms whirl the same swirling motion. The first set have the right arm whirl clockwise and left arms counterclockwise, with the hands meeting in the center. Second set whirl the opposite direction.
3. breath normal

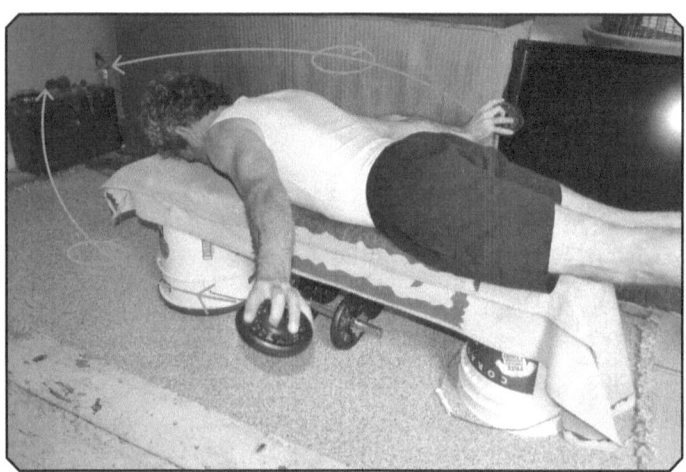

## 5. Whirling Modified Back Fly

The Whirling Modified Back Fly completes a balanced workout. It develops the muscles of the upper back and shoulders. The trapezius and rhomboids gets worked thoroughly. The deltoid, and triceps also get an additional work due to the whirling motion. The erector spinae, (muscle along the spine], help hole the back strait and get a nice workout also.

A. Lie on your chest on the bench and hold each dumbbells at the sides of your hips. Arms should be slightly arched

B. Bring both dumbbells forward while whirling your arms until they are close to be fully extended pass your head. Then bring the arms back down to you hips while whirling. It's as if you were to move your arms from down your sides to over your head, while whirling them. The whirls should be about 6-inch diameter and 4 to 5 whirls up and the same down. The whirl comes from the shoulder joint and not the elbow or wrist. Right arm performs clockwise whirls while the left arm in counterclockwise for first set and the reverse whirl for the second set.

C. Breathing should be normal as long as you don't hold your breath.

CHAPTER **2**

# GRAVITY YOGA

The second groups of exercises are a little bit yoga; a little bit me, and a little bit Bruce Lee. I hybridized the three of them. These exercises contain no massage, but when done correctly, it can produce unmatched relaxation. This is vital to athleticisms and health in general. These are the best exercises for correcting scoliosis and any imbalances you have. This is excellent for body sculpting and getting the shape you desire. Gravity Yoga aligns the body in ways that any yoga or stretching can not. All thanks to the use of gravity. This is a very low-keyed exercise and can be performed by mostly anyone. However some people that have high blood pressure sometimes have problems whenever the feet are raised above the head. Once again, always ask your doctor before starting ant exercise.

Gravity is the reason so many people have bad posture. This causes many types of back and spinal problems. Gravity weighs us down, pulling the head and shoulders down, crushing our joints. It accentuates curves in our posture, which limits athletic ability at best, and cripples at worst. These curves in the spine get worst, as we get older. Sore and tight muscles always accompany these curves. Well, good news. My stretches harness the power of gravity, to heal those very same muscles that gravity has stressed. I use gravity to force muscles to stretch that can't be accomplished as well any other way.

The idea here is to lie on the floor with your feet strait up a wall or on a chair. In this position gravity forces the back flat against the floor. Here is how to correct these problems. You will complete a series of stretches in this position of lying on the floor. The legs and feet go up a wall or up on a chair. The wall is strongly preferred over the chair. Gravity eventually takes over and forces your spine to relax and align. Gravity is needed to overcome those shorten, stiff muscles that prevent proper posture. Proper poster is paramount when performing these stretches. This should be your main focus. These stretches require breathing correctly while holding a pose.

Short carpeting or wood floor is fine as long as it is not cold. I feel a mirror on the ceiling is almost necessary. The mirror can be attached quite cheaply with some eye hooks and fishing line. Be careful and attach the mirror securely. Get a professional or someone that knows what they're doing, You don't want a mirror falling on you. You can wear spandex shorts and shirt and tight, slightly small and undersized is preferred. You can see so much more of the body in the mirror this way. Looking at subtle difference is very important. Balance is everything.

The first step is to lie with your hands rotated out and down your sides. Take notice of your body's centerline. Are both sides equal? A strait line should follow up the spine and through the center of the back of the head. Is it strait? And how do I move or shift to do to make it strait? What areas don't come in contact with the floor? For many people it's the lower back and the neck that resist touching the floor. These areas that are raised off the floor are usually where tight muscles are located. That's why you can't get them to touch the floor. The muscles are so tight that they do not allow the spine to straitened and lengthen. As you perform these exercises, try to bring them flat on the floor. I am constantly rolling my head forward with my hand enabling my neck to lie flat on the floor. The goal here is to get the entire spine to lie flat with every vertebra touching the floor.

In this position, breathe in a pattern of 7 to 8 fast breaths then hold on the inhale for 12 seconds then exhaled quickly. If you prefer to just lay there relaxed and perform deep breathing, that is great! In fact I recommend it. Deep breathing where you breath in for about 4 seconds, hold for a second, and breathe out for 2 seconds, is very therapeutic and relaxing. This type of meditative breathing benefits ever system in the body. But for active stretching, it is not appropriate because of the large amount of oxygen and energy required performing Gravity Yoga. This breathing should be with the diaphragm, in other words, breath with your stomach and not your upper back. Lying flat helps to isolate the diaphragm and prevent back breathing. The ribs should be expanded and spread apart and the spine should be as close to the floor as possible. Breathing with the diaphragm is proper breathing. Most people are back breathers, using their back and chest cavity to draw air into the lungs. This is wrong and can lead to posture problems and curvature of the spine. This is probable the main reason for spinal curvature as we age.

Studies have show that whenever you stretch, it should be held for at least 12 seconds or no benefit will occur. All muscles being stretch must be held for at least 12 seconds, if they are to be effective. I prefer to hold a stretch for minutes rather than seconds

Muscle spasms are not that uncommon after performing these stretches. Sometimes you will notice that when you stand up after performing theses exercises, you will feel spasms in some of the muscles in your back, but don't worry. They only last for a few minutes. These spasms occur to the muscles that are forced to contract for extended periods as a result of lying on the floor. These spasms are usually not a bad thing. It's just week muscles reacting to being used and strengthened. These spasms usually occur in the areas of the back that have an outward curve. These outward curves are surrounded by week, elongated muscles. By lying on the floor, the week muscles in that area are forced to contract and get shorter. In essence, those week muscles are becoming stronger and shorter, and that's what you want. And those spasms just mean you are giving those week muscles a good workout. These spasm usually cause a person to stand erect and in better posture.

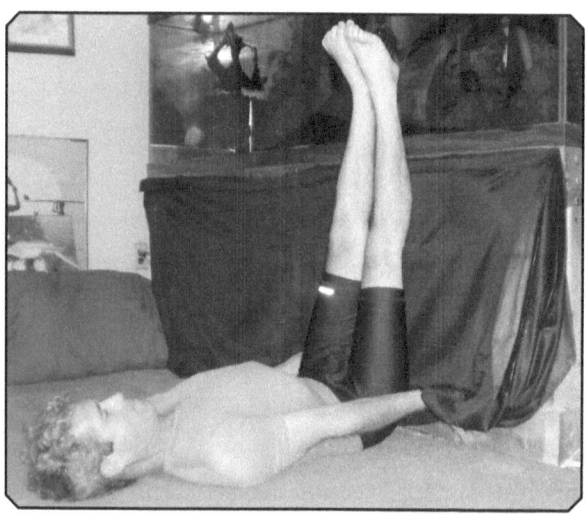

Let's sum this up. You're lying on the floor, trying to straiten your spine, and breathing as described. Now are you ready to start stretching on top of all that? It takes some concentration but I know you can do it! Pay careful attention to your balance. Always ask yourself questions like, why can I raise one arm higher than the other, or why do my hips seam twisted and what do I do to correct this? Pay attention to all the noises to joints and bones aligning and how it feels. Pay attention to areas and muscles that may fell stiff or hurt from the floors pressure.

These stretches are great for everyone. The old love it because it's regenerating. The young like it because it will change the shape of your body and improve everything you do.

A guy I worked with had a son that applied for a job. They gave him a physical, and then denied him the job because he had a large curvature of the spine (scoliosis). They were considering surgery and other invasive techniques to correct this. I explained that if there wasn't an immediate concern to correct this problem, then maybe he should try some stretches from Gravity Yoga. Two years latter he has almost totally correct the scoliosis. He reapplied and was hired by the very same company that denied previously.

These stretches are designed to increase the range of motion in all your joints. I like to call these stretches reverse impact because they elongate your body, not compress it. Now let's stretch!

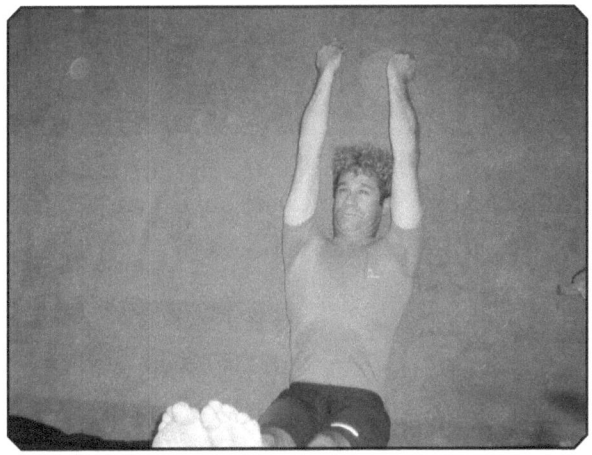

(A) 1. Raise both arms overhead as high as possible, rotate palms facing in, breathe as described and keep your back flat. The ribs should be equally spread apart, if one arm doesn't go as high as the other, or you feel you are deficient in a particular area, spend more time and concentration on it. Everyone must work on his or her own individual weakness and strengths that are completely unique to oneselve. Therefore no one should have the same workout. And workouts should change depending on what is needed.

2. Rotate arms out, hold fore 1 min.

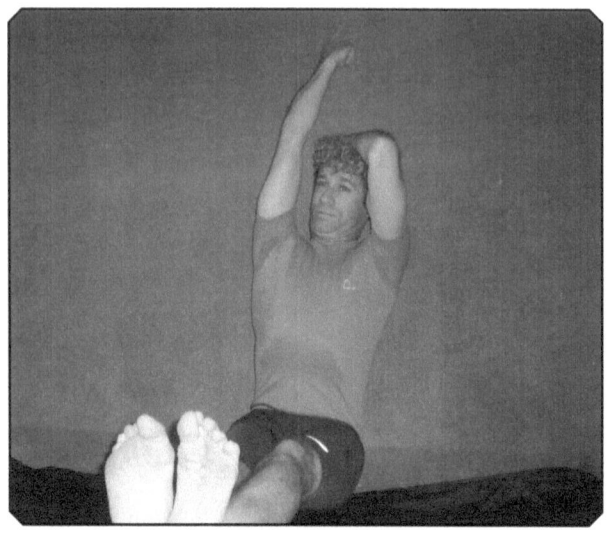

3. Right arm, Rotated in 30 sec. Rotate out 30 sec. see pic above

4. Left arm, rotate in 30 sec. Rotate out 30 sec

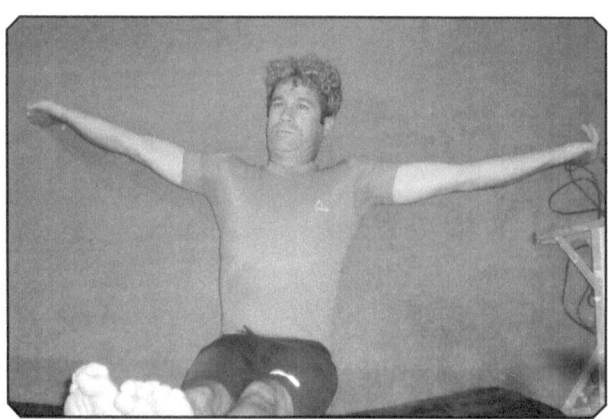

5. Repeat sequence with arms held laterally at 90 to 120 degrees. Pic above

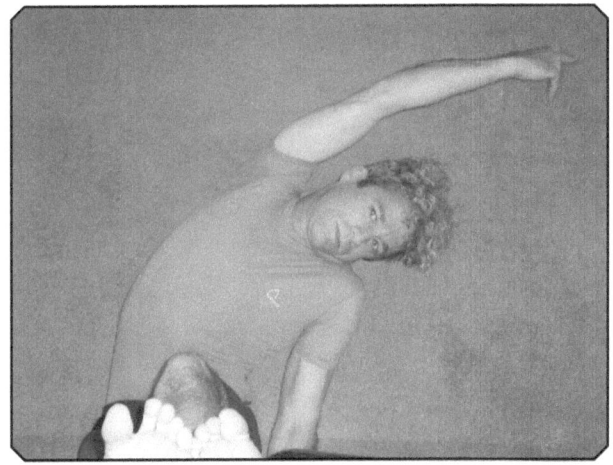

(B) 1. Right side stretch. This really stretches out the latissimus dorsi (lats) and all those little muscles between the ribs (intercostals). This also provides great flexibility of the spine. Rotate arms in and out fore 30 sec. If it helps to cross the right leg over the left leg, than do it.

2   Do the left side same as the right side. If one side doesn't stretch as much as the other side, than work more on the stiffer side more. Try to gain balance in the right and left sides.

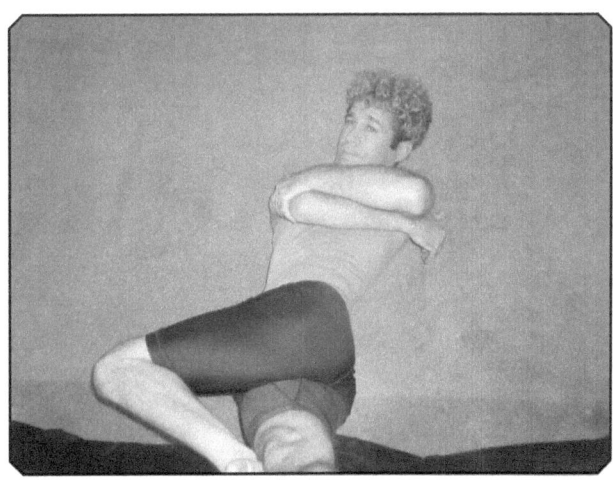

(C) 1. Pull your right arm across the chest with left arm, pulling the scapula away from the spine. The key is to pull the shoulder blade (scapula) as far from the spine as possible. The hips are twisted and off the floor, with the aid of the legs. With the hips off the floor most of the body's weight can be focus on the shoulder blade area. The muscles around the scapula receive lots of stress and are very hard to stretch. By allowing gravity to force your body's weight on that area, will aid in separating the shoulder blade away from the spine stretching those tight muscles. By applying pressure to the shoulder blade area not only stretches those muscles, but the pressure further increasing the stretch with a deep pressure massage. It's a double whammy: where as you are relaxing tense muscle with a great stretch and a deep pressure massage, all in one exercise. These muscles in the shoulder blade area are such a problem because there really isn't an effective stretch that will alleviate this type of muscular tension, till now.

Hold this stretch for 1 min. This stretch is designed to stretch the upper and middle trapizius muscles (traps), and those little muscle that surround the scapula. This also gives a great twisting like stretch to the spine. This is very important to golfers. Once this stretch is mastered, you will hit the golf ball further and more accurate.

2. Do the left side the same as right side. Pay attention if one side stretches' easier than the other and work on your weaknesses.

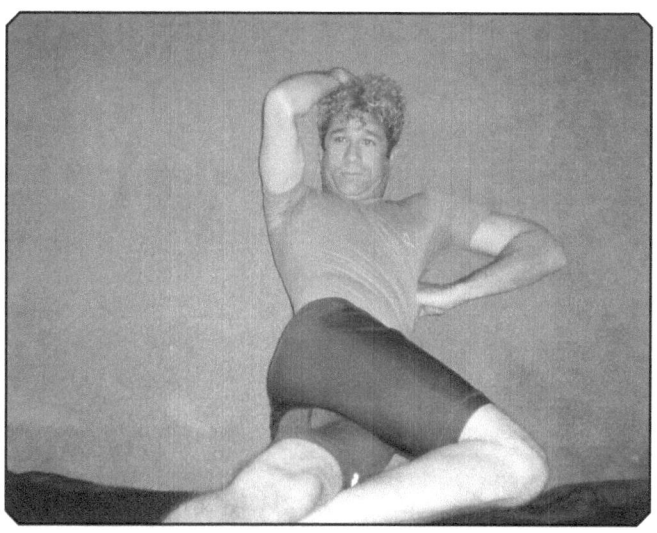

3. This stretch can be performed with the arms in what I call the chicken wing position, as seen here. This allows for a greater stretch to the muscles around the shoulder blades (scapula) and the deltoid muscle.

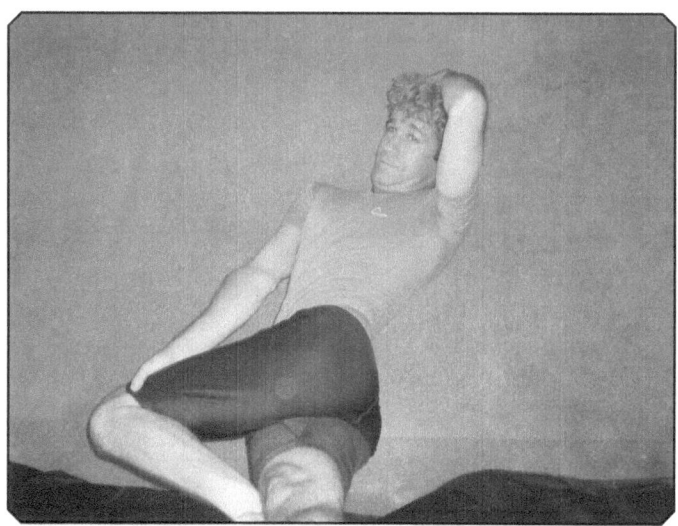

(D) 1. Right arm down your side or on left leg and roll of your body's weight on to the right shoulder blade. Pulling the head away from right shoulder with your left hand increases the stretch of the upper trapizius muscle. This is similar to the previous exercise where the hips are twisted and off the floor. The traps are where so many people have tense stiff muscles from carrying the weight of the arms all day. This stretch will help people with rounded shoulders. It also gives a great spine stretch that is of value to golfers or any other athlete. Hold for 1min.

2.  Do the left side same as right. Be aware of any differences between the right side and the left.

(E) End like you started, with your hands strait down you sides and breathing correctly, rotate arms in and out. Take notice of how easy it is to breath and how much straighter your back is. Even when standing, your shoulders feel lighter and you more comfortable.

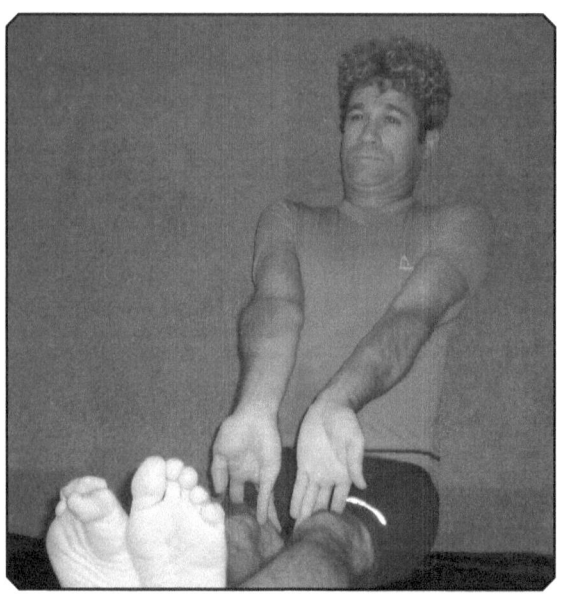

(F) Be inventive. Go over your weaknesses. Hold your arms in various positions to invent new stretches. Try both arms down at the sides, and hands on the knees to stretch the hamstrings.

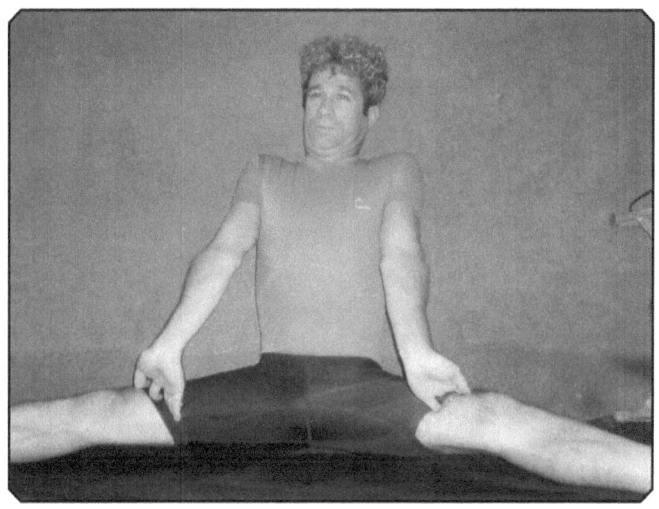

Increase your range of motion. Now try these exercise with your legs straddled or split apart. This really helps to free up the lower back and hips. This also a great groin and hamstring stretch.

**Complimentary exercises**.

Now that you spent at least 30 min. to an hour on the floor you are ready for the second half of Gravity Yoga. These stretches are to compliment and add balance to those stretches that were performed while on the floor. All are with normal breathing with diaphragm.

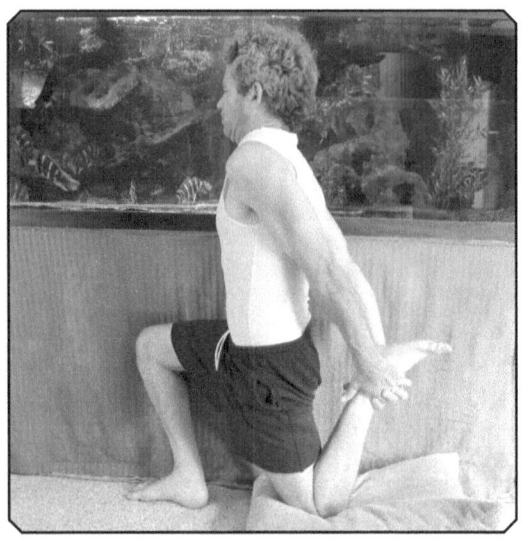

(A) 1. First thing is to stretch the quadriceps that had become short as a result of your legs being up the wall. This stretch is very important to do after if you completed the previous exercises. Right knee down and hold the right ankle with both hands and lean forward, forcing the right hip forward. Hold for 30 sec. To 2 min. keep back and neck strait. It may help to lean against a wall when doing this.

2. Do the Left side
3. Repeat (A) 1and 2

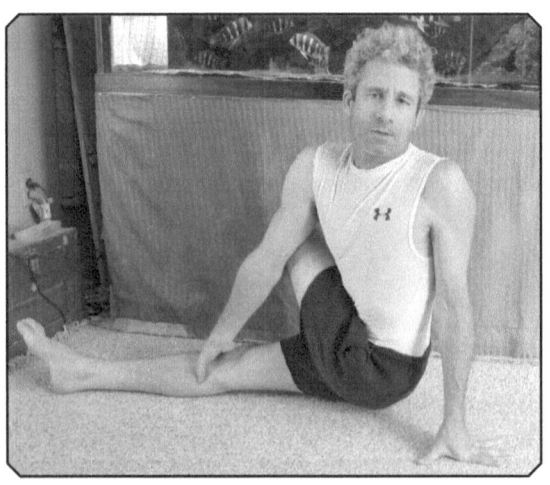

(B) 1. Next is the common twist the spine stretch, cross your legs and raise your right knee. Place right arm on left knee and left hand on the floor behind you and twist. Keep spine strait up and down but twisted as your shoulders turn one way and your hips the other way. Hold for 1 min.

2. Do the left side.

3. Repeat (C) 1 and 2

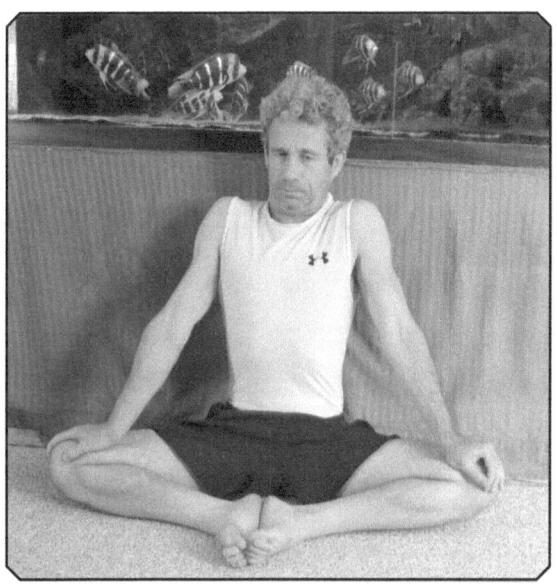

(C) Groin stretch. In a seated position, push knees down with hands. Hold for 1min. It helps to lean your back against a wall to keep back strait.

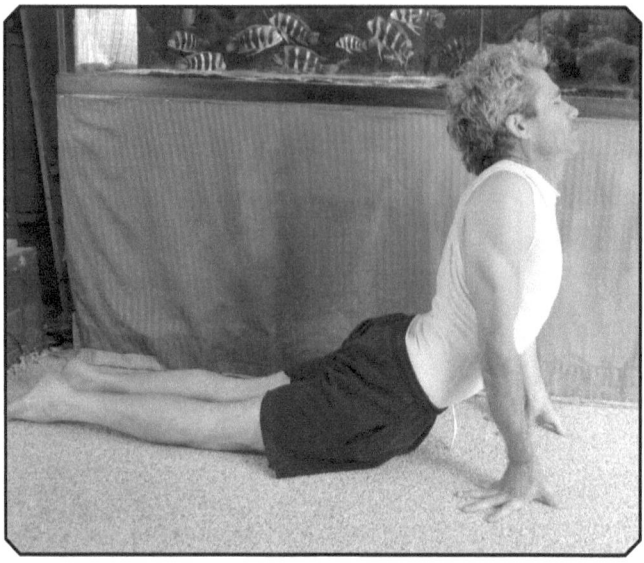

(E) 1. The cat revised. Lying facing the floor, arms strait and under the shoulders and hips on the floor. I like to roll my head and shoulders around. Hold for 30sec.

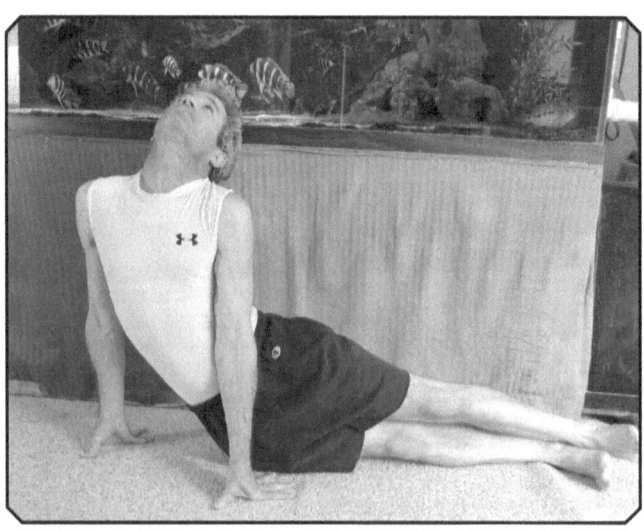

2. Roll on to right side and arch back downward allowing gravity to assist you. Hold for 30sec.

3. Do the left side

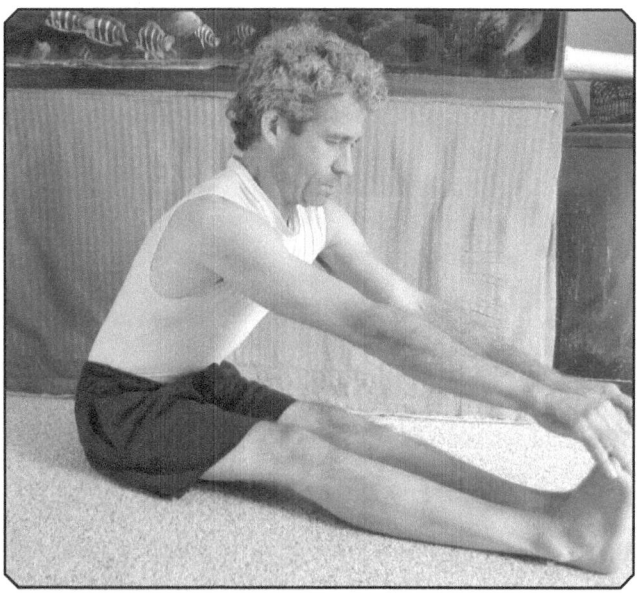

(F) This is the classic touch your toes stretch for the hamstrings. Keep back strait, shoulders down, and if you grab your toes, you can stretch the calf muscles out as well.

# Chapter 3

# THE COACH POTATO

This massage is for almost everyone. And is far less extreme and intense than The Ripper. But can be just as rewarding. As always, ask your doctor before starting any exercise and please read the list of contraindications at the end of the chapter.

The average chair is a killer!!!! People that live sedentary lifestyles, sitting down for 8 to 12 hours a day will shorten their lifespan significantly. It has been proven in many scientific studies. And who would of thought that having a desk job would kill you sooner than many labor-intensive jobs. Well its true. but not with my chair technique. While watching TV in the comfort of your favorite chair, you can get all the effects of a great massage, rid yourself of pain, burn calories, and flatten your stomach. And what could be more convenient then sitting in your chair while watching the TV? In other words, if you have time for TV, you have time for The Coach Potato.

Massage is usually not considered exercise because it usually requires little effort. I however, place my massage into the world of exercise because the person who is receiving the massage is the same person giving the massage. As you give this massage, the core muscles will be getting a good workout also. All the muscles needed for correct posture will be affected, including the abdominals. Yes it is possible to develop a six-pack while watching TV.

A young apprentice who had a wife and many children, ask me what he could do to relax and just release some stress. The only problem is that the only time he has to himself is before dinner and that's when he watches The News. I informed him about the couch potato. One week later he' told me his family thinks he's crazy zigzagging back in fourth in his chair, but he didn't care. He told me he has never felt better and now he's sleeping through the night even when the baby is crying. His wife does not like that but he does.

Many elderly and people that are not in great shape love the couch potato because it's easy to perform, convenient and has big results.

I know I said this stuff before but I need to reinforce it, Now there are many types of massage chairs and other gimmicks on the market but none of them can do what you can do for your self. You will have the distinct advantage of knowing exactly where the tight spots are because they are hard, lumpy and feel sore. Some of muscles are so sensitive that the slightest touch sends you in pain. There is no therapist and certainly not a mechanical massage chair that knows your body like you do. Therefore self -massage can be the best form of massage. These techniques have no end, for it is an ongoing process that evolves around one's unique needs throughout life.

Self-massage is also free. There isn't a therapist collecting a bill. There isn't any wasted time traveling. There isn't the high cost of a massage chair that runs on electricity. It's just you getting an awesome massage, free of charge, any time that you want. All my exercises are low budget.

At this time I would like to briefly state some of the benefits of massage. There are many books on the subject but here are the basics.

1. Massage tones and relieves sore stiff muscles. It relaxes spastic muscles.
2. Massage improves circulation, getting nutrients into the cells and removing waist.

3. Massage increases blood supply to the skin, keeping it functioning normal and looking young.

4. Massage increases blood to the brain and nerves helping to alleviate stress.

5. Massage increases lymph circulation, which helps to eliminate waist and stimulate the immune system.

6. Massage aids digestion, relaxing intestinal muscles and improving kidneys and liver function.

7. Simply put, massage is awesome!

This is what is needed for the couch potato besides the TV and comfy chair. You will need a one inch thick wood plank a proximately 18in. by 30in. It should be long enough to extend beyond your head when it is placed on the back of the hair. This plank can be removed when not performing a massage. The chair should lean back slightly but not in a reclined position. A stool works ideally also.

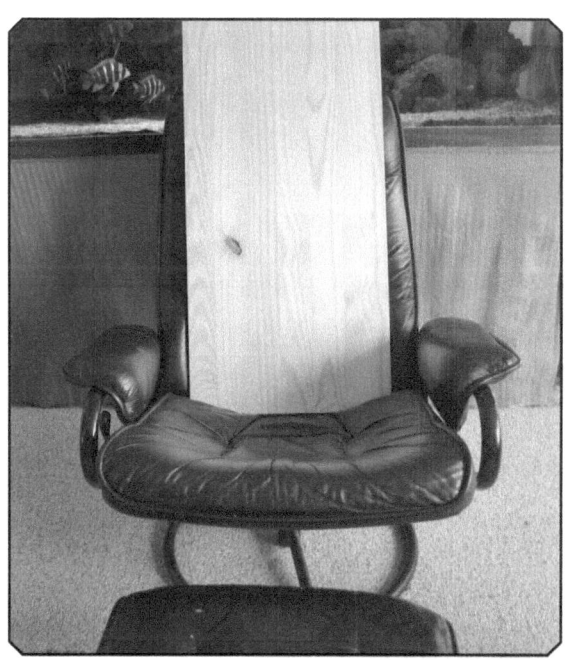

You will need a lacrosse ball for this exercise. You may need to scuff the ball up with sandpaper so it does not slip around making the movement of the ball difficult to control.

I also recommend the use of a spandex shirt or at least a long cotton t-shirt that can be tucked under your butt when sitting. This helps to keep the ball from grabbing the fabric in shirt. Be careful not to chaff or irritate your skin when performing self-massage. Be aware of what's happening. If an area gets irritated, move to another area or stop the massage for a day or two. Slowly work your way into theses exercises, and don't over do it.

It is very important to stay hydrated and drink plenty of water. Part of massage is the ability to remove wastes from your cells by flushing them with water. Water is key for removing toxins. Water also brings nutrients to the cell, aids in digestion, lubricates joints and aids in athletic performance.

Make sure you read the list of contraindications ( when you shouldn't receive a massage at the end of this chapter.

The basic idea behind the couch potato is the ball is placed between you and the plank on the back of the chair. You sit in the chair as normal but you move and wiggle around in a manor that rolls the massage ball up both sides of the back in a zig zag pattern. Your legs, hips, arms and shoulders facilitate this motion. All your core muscles will be in use but you won't even realize it because you will be watching TV. The use of a footstool is recommended. Yes, you even get to put your feet up. See

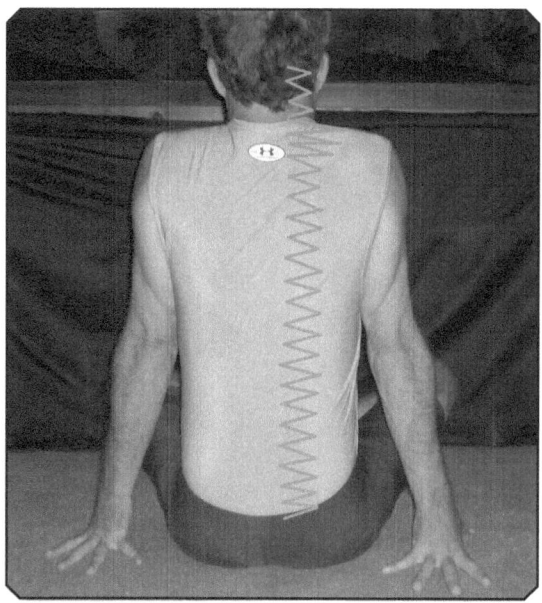

In accordance with Swedish massage and with regards to blood flow direction, you begin on the lower back and proceed up towards the head.

Make no mistake, this in not the same massage as you get from massage chairs. Once mastered, my massage will out perform any massage chair or even massage therapist. And it's free!!! And it burns calories and flattens your stomach. No massage chair can promise you that.

Start with the right side first. Begin low on the back, possibly hitting the upper gluteus muscles. Then proceed up towards the head. Do not roll over your vertebrae or scapula. Move your body from side to side in order to get the ball to zigzag up the back. Zigzag as much as feel necessary. 30 is a good number, to make it up your head

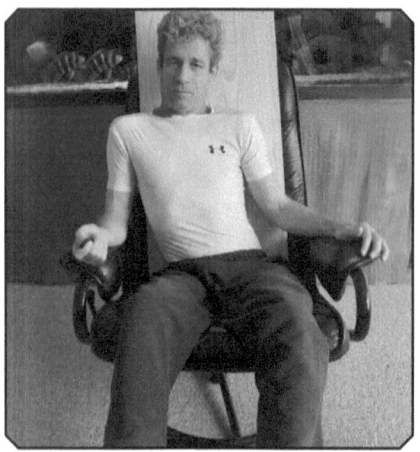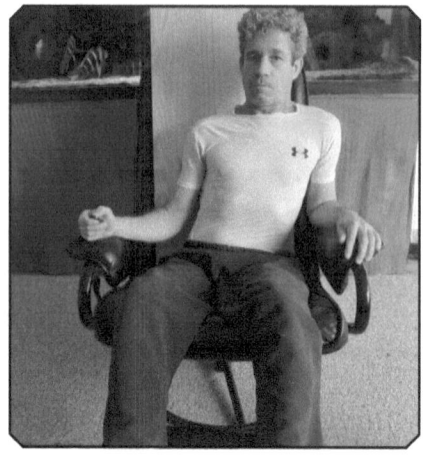

Attempt the right side then the left. Try it for a half an hour. Practice makes perfect and you will master it. Sometimes you will have to adjust the ball with a hand in order to stay on pattern or stay on a particularly tense area. By keeping your neck and back as strait as possible, this will place those tense muscles on a slight stretch, greatly aiding the effects of the massage. I advise to grab the back of the head when working the neck and head area. Be careful not to pull your hair out. The ball can grab hair and the use of a spandex bathing cap eliminates this problem. Grabbing the back of the head and extending the neck will aid in the stretching of these muscles and help keep control of the ball. Remember, the harder the ball and the harder you press the deeper the massage is. Always start soft and slow, then proceed to dig in and apply pressure. Some muscles may be so sore and tight that the ball will barely roll over them. In fact, you will hear everything from little crackles to deep thumps as the ball attempts to roll over stiff muscles. Theses noises fade as muscles relax and the massage proceeds.

Certain muscles will be so sore that even the slightest pressure will hurt and cause pain. But somehow it feels good to press on and work that stiff muscle free. Occasionally a stiff muscle will relax suddenly and that is what I like to call a musclegasm A truly relaxed muscle will be as soft and smooth as silk. It will take time, but you will notice large results your first time. Practice makes perfect. You may experience additional muscle soreness after completion of this exercise, but that is common with deep pressure massage and will fade as you progress. I have heard this soreness described as a "good hurt". ALWAYS START THE COUCH POTATOE SOFT AND SLOW. Only do a little at first. You need to know how much pressure your body can take. Then, in future exercises slowly apply more pressure. If skin becomes too iterated, let adequate time for healing. I can't stress this enough, but pay attention to what your body is telling you.

It is with hope, that once you have mastered the couch potato you will attempt the chapter called "The Ripper". The Ripper is a much more intense self-massage with huge results.

## CONTRAINDICATIONS

Contraindication means that it may not be advisable to massage yourself performing the ripper or even the couch potato. I caution you, when in doubt, always refer to a doctor. DO YOUR BODY NO HARM. Here's the list of when not to give yourself or receive a massage.

1. Massage, especially deep pressure, will make a cold or flu worse. A fever is definitely a no go situation.
2. Any acute inflammation like arthritis, neuritis, or dermatitis. Be cautious to stay away from those areas, if a massage is given at all.
3. Any inflammation from tissue damage. Stay off the discolored, swollen areas.
4. Any visible bacteria infections, (pus)
5. Osteoporosis (bone deterioration) or any frail, old people
6. Anywhere there are varicose veins
7. Swollen, painful veins known as phlebitis or any kind of circulatory abnormality

8. High blood pressure is not for the ripper, but maybe the couch potato. If done lightly, massage will aid in lowering it blood pressure

9. If you are extremely tired or fatigued

10. Any kind of skin problem

11. Scoliosis (crooked spine). Massage must be given with extreme care. Gravity Yoga will help this condition.

12. Any kind of disease or condition see you doctor.

## CHAPTER 4

# THE RIPPER

This is an extreme exercise yielding huge results. The Ripper can be dangerous to perform, and You should always ask your doctor before starting this and all exercise. Please read my list of contraindications at the end of this chapter.

I named this self-massage technique, The Ripper, because it tears into the toughest muscle knots, with extreme prejudice. The Ripper will unlock the most spastic of muscles. This is the most efficient way to get, and give, the deepest massage ever! You will learn about your body, and discover where exactly those tense spots are and relieve them. You will learn how to pinpoint problems through personal bio-feedback (what feels good and what doesn't) and learn to correct those problems. You will gain freedom of movement that you never had. You will become the athlete you never were.

This is really one of my favorite exercises. It's fun and you receive immediate results. Lets face it, exercises like lifting weights, running, riding the elliptical machine or bike, suck. Sure you fell good afterwards because of the endorphins, and you do it because of the benefits, but it sucks. The ripper is fun to do! No matter what level of game or sport you're in, the ripper will increase it. Top athletes pay attention!!!

Unlike most other types of massages, The Ripper burns many calories therefore I categorize this self-massage as exercise. You get a great workout and the best massage ever.

Besides getting an awesome massage, The Ripper will work the abdominal muscles extensively. Why waste time doing 100 to 1000 sit ups a day when you can spend that same time getting a better abdominal work with the best massage ever? You will never have to do another sit up again and feel great for it.

A roofer came to me with sever neck and shoulder pain. He could not lift his left arm. He was about to lose his job because he could not keep up with the young guys. This guy would carry a 90-pound roll of roofing material up a ladder many times a day. The left arm would hold the material; wile the right arm grabbed the ladder. Just by looking at him I could tell that his upper trapezius muscle on the left side was tight and short. After feeling the tenseness of the muscle I was correct. It was a typical over worked muscle syndrome. The answer was easy. He needed to relax and stretch that muscle out. I advised him to lay on the lacrosse ball in that area, move the ball around and give the upper trap muscle a good deep pressure massage. He came back to me the next day and told me that he could now raise his arm. This is something he hasn't been able to do in many years, and his back pain was gone also. He is now off all the medications and stop going to Physical therapy. No one was able to give this roofer a deep pressure massage that was required to free up this large extra thick muscle. To be honest, I doubt anyone could give him a deep enough massage, except for him self. This roofer weighed well over 200 lbs. He would place all his bodies weight on that lacrosse ball for 20 minutes. To this day he still calls me filled with gratitude. 7 years latter he is still pain free and working.

If you doubt me, just take that lacrosse ball and roll it around under your feet for 5 minutes. Then compare that foot to the other foot that didn't receive a massage. Big difference!

Golfers really seem to notice the effects of the ripper. It's because so much of a golfers swing relies on the flexibility of the back to create a large range of motion. This increase in the range of motion directly corresponds to hitting the ball further and more accurately. Get in on the secret of The Ripper before the competition does.

Now that I have you all hyped up, I have to warn that the ripper has to begin slowly and with extreme caution. Muscles and skin need time to adapt. The couch potatoes should be mastered before attempting the ripper unless you are in good shape. In addition, performing the chapter called, Gravity Yoga, will help you warm up for the ripper. Please read list of contraindications or when it may not be advisable for massage. The ripper should not be attempted by anyone with any medical condition including old age and always ask your doctor first before starting any exercise or diet program. This is found at the end of this chapter. When performing The Ripper, one or two balls are place between your back and the floor. Tennis balls can be used but they tend not to work well. They flatten out under your body weight and won't roll. Lacrosse balls should be used and are ideal for deep tissue massage. You may need to take sandpaper to the surface of the lacrosse ball. Sometimes when you buy these balls they have a slippery surface and that make the ball hard to control. Overweight individuals can use rubber softballs. Short carpeting is preferred but wood or tile will work as long as the ball doesn't slide around. You move the ball by moving your body. Wearing a spandex shirt will help with chaffing but any shirt will have a tendency to grab on to the ball so the tighter the shirt and pants the better. Bicycle pants work well also. Tight cloths (spandex) works best because the ball has a tendency to grab loose fitting cloths. Spandex pants will help keep the shirt tucked in and tight. This will help prevent the ball from grabbing onto the shirt. This can be a problem if not wearing the proper attire. Be careful when performing some of these exercises that the ball doesn't grab your hair and pull it out. The use of a spandex bathing cap can eliminate this problem.

Chaffing is to be expected at first, so if an area gets too raw just work on another area or stop. Wait a couple of days, and apply less or no pressure or to that area. Your skin will adapt in time and will have a healthier texture. At one point I used a golf ball and I wore no shirt. A mirror on the ceiling is strongly advised for the biofeedback. I cannot stress this enough. It is important that you see what your body is doing and are you performing in a balanced manor.

Now there are many types of massage chairs and other gimmicks on the market but none of them can do what you can do for your self. You will have the distinct advantage of knowing exactly where the tight spots are because they are hard, lumpy and feel sore. Some of muscles are so sensitive that the slightest touch sends you in pain. There is no therapist and certainly not a mechanical massage chair that knows your body like you do. Therefore self -massage can be the best form of massage. These techniques have no end point, for it is an ongoing process that evolves around one's unique needs throughout life.

Self-massage is also free. There isn't a therapist collecting a bill. There isn't any wasted time traveling. There isn't the high cost of a massage chair that runs on electricity. It's just you getting an awesome massage, free of charge, any time that you want. All my exercises are low budget.

At this time I would like to briefly state some of the benefits of massage. There are many books on the subject but here are the basics.

1. Massage tones and relieves sore stiff muscles. It relaxes spastic muscles.
2. Massage improves circulation, getting nutrients into the cells and removing waist.
3. Massage increases blood supply to the skin, keeping it functioning normal and looking young.
4. Massage increases blood to the brain and nerves helping to alleviate stress.

5. Massage increases lymph circulation, which helps to eliminate waist and stimulate the immune system.
6. Massage aids digestion, relaxing intestinal muscles and improving kidneys and liver function.
7. Simply put, massage is awesome!

Once again, staying hydrated is paramount. Drink plenty of water even if you have to urinate every 20 minutes because the ripper forces water and nutrients in and out of the cells quickly. This massage facilitates the removal of toxins from the cells. So every time you urinate, it is a good time to drink more water. Water also aids in digestion, lubricates joints and transportation of nutrients to the cells. Hydration will be discussed in the Nutrition chapter.

You will be amazed at the noises that occur while performing these exercises. You will hear loud thumps as the balls rolls over tight spastic muscles. You will hear vertebrae and joints pop, crackle and snap as they shift into alignment as corresponding muscles relax. You do not roll the balls over the vertebrae. Your doctor or chiropractor should do any manipulation to the spine.

I explain The Ripper in easy to follow massages to various areas of the body. It is best to start at the area furthest from the heart and work towards it. That would be the gluteus and sacral area is the starting point. So here is the quick overview for The Ripper. I know it seems complicated at first but it follows a very logical order and will be learned quickly. This can be completed in 20 minutes but I prefer to do it for an hour. That's how much I like it.

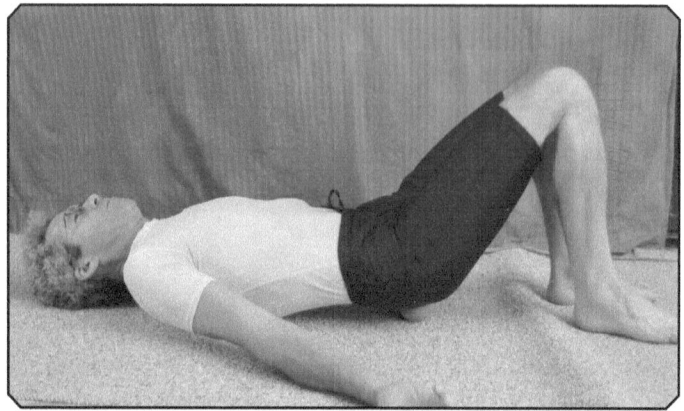

1   <u>Massage the Gluteus and sacral area with 2 balls</u>. Lying on the floor, knees bent with feet close to butt, arms at sides, all but your hips are in contact with the floor. Raise the hips of the floor with the aid of the legs and contacting the abdominal muscles. The balls are placed on equal sides of the hip. Vey little pressure is applied to the balls with most of the weight is on the legs. You don't want to put to much weight on the balls. This is a sensitive area so don't apply to much pressure on the balls. Gently twist, wiggle and roll your hips around. What ever you have to do to get those balls to roll around to massage in the hip area. Gently roll over the sacrum, tailbone and rim of the hip. The upper portion of the gluteus muscle can be massage with more pressure but most of the weight will be resting on your legs. Light pressure is all that is needed. This should only take 30 seconds or so. Or how ever long you like it. With all my exercise if you feel the need to stay on an area, do it. Everyone has his or her own individual needs.

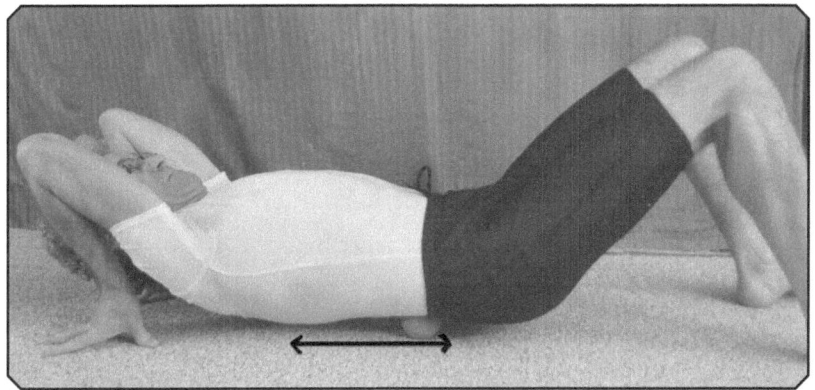

2   Massage the lower back with 2 balls. Lying on the floor, knees bent with feet close to butt, arms extended overhead with palms on the floor. The balls are placed on each side of the lower back just above the crest of the hip. The body is lifted off the floor with the aid of the legs and arms with some of the body's weight resting on the balls. The arms and legs dictate how much weight is on the balls. The balls are rolled up and down each side of the spine from the hip crest to the middle of the back somewhere just below the shoulder blades. Its really not that important how far you roll up the back, but this should be accomplished with one smooth movement up and down. For most people this about half way up the back before they have to start moving the hands and feet to much to accomplish a smooth movement. The feet or the hands should not have to move much. The more floor space you have available, the better because you tend to move around quit a bit. If you don't have much floor space readjust your position if you start drifting off the available floor space. The arms and legs will lift most of your body's weight, with little pressure on the balls. As you progress more and more pressure can be applied to get a deeper and deeper massage for those large tense muscles of the lower back. Many people get to the point where all of the body's weight is focused on the balls and the arms and legs just move the body up and down, Take notice of all the

noises that occur and how they make your body feel. Fell and hear the vertebrae as they shift into alignment, the thumps as the ball rolls over thick muscles. Take notice of how thick and stiff the lower back muscle feel and how much more relaxed they become as you progress. The goal is to keep the balls in sync and parallel to each other as they roll up and down your back. This can be difficult at first but readjust the balls as often as needed. Do not roll over the spine or the crest of the hip. Do this exercise anywhere from 10 to 50 times or however long you like it. Be careful and don't let the balls chaff you.

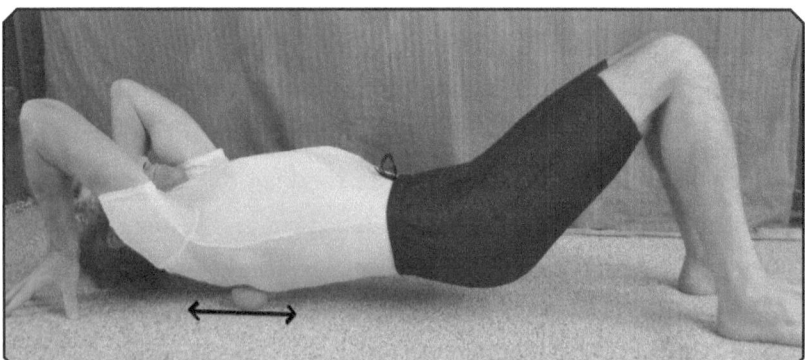

3   <u>Massage the upper back and shoulder area with 2 balls</u>. Lying on the floor in the same position as exercise 2 the balls are placed in the upper back region along the spine. The balls are rolled up and down the spine from below the scapula along the upper back to about the beginning of the neck, in the same manner and position as exercise 2. Once this position is mastered then you can try this with the arms folded across the chest. This aids the massage by exposing more muscles and providing a deeper massage because the arms are no longer holding your body weight and more pressure is applied to the balls. Don't roll over the spine or the scapula. Keep the balls parallel to each other. One smooth movement up and down and

the legs or arms should not have to move much. Try to get all those thick muscle that surround the scapula. Pay attention to the noises and as vertebrae adjust and how the deep thumps as the ball rolls over stiff muscles. Once again, start off with light pressure but once you are accustomed you can really apply the pressure to those tight areas. Don't be afraid to just stay on a particular stiff area and just lean heavily on that ball for minutes in one place. Many times that is what's needed to relax a spastic muscle and the shoulder area seems to have lots of this. It's musclegasm city, Do this exercise 10 to 50 times.

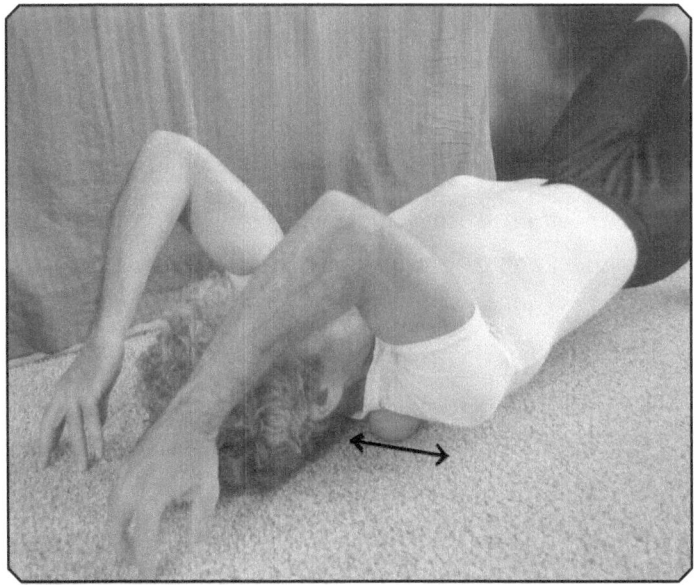

4   Massage the trapezius (top of shoulders) muscles with 2 balls. Lying on the floor in the same position as exercise 2 and 3, the balls are placed under the trapezius muscle on the upper shoulder and lower neck area just above the scapula. It's a small area, but that little triangle of muscle holds a great deal of stress in most people. Instead or moving the body in an up and down movement like in previous

exercises, here the movement is a side to side, kind of rocking motion so that the balls roll along the tops of the shoulders. Don't roll over the spine or the top of the scapula. Go back and fourth 10 to 50 times.

---

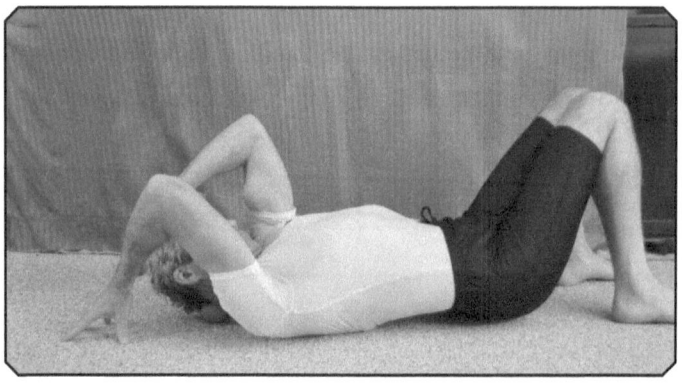

5   <u>Massage the neck and scalp with 1 ball</u>. It can't be done with 2 balls. The body position is the same as the previous exercise except that most of the body is resting on the floor and supporting weight. one arm is used to support the body's weight and the other arm is placed on the back top of the head. This is done to support the head and keep the neck inline and in position. Try to get your head to roll forward placing the chin to the chest. If you are massaging the right side of the neck use the left hand to slightly grabbing and pulling the head to the left while lowering the right shoulder. This will stretch upper trapezius muscles in the back of the neck area, which aids the massage. The hand that's on the floor will aid in the little bit of movement that is required. The body is on the floor except the head. The ball is rolled several times up and down the neck, from the upper shoulder area to the base of the skull and never touching the vertebrae. Then zigzag patterns a few times. The zigzag patterns are designed to strum the muscles, like a guitar, that run along the

spine. This will make load-thumping noises when done correctly. Go up and down the necks only a few times then do the other side. These muscles relax quickly to massage and usually not much time is required on this area.

------------------------------------------------------------

6   Massage the Gluteus and sacral area with 2 balls. Repeat exercise 1

------------------------------------------------------------

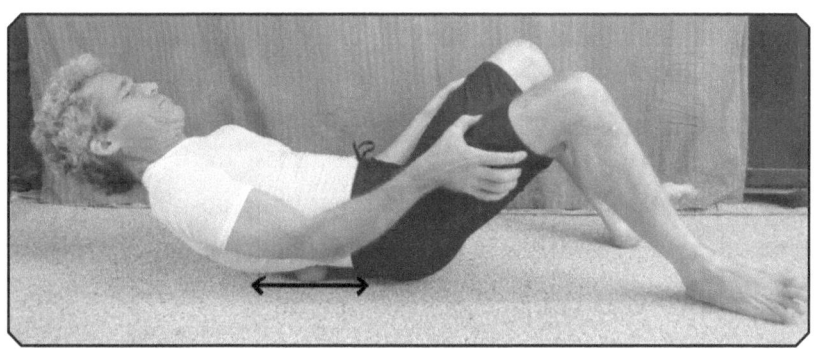

7   Massage the lower back in the crunch position. With 2 balls Lying on the floor with knees bent and feet close to the butt, abdominals are contacted and upper back is off the floor. This will place the muscles of the lower back on a slight stretch, greatly aiding the effects of the massage. This is like the position of a crunch sit-up with the body resting all of it's weight on the balls and the legs. The arms are at side with hands gripping the upper thighs or buttocks. The arms are helping support the abdominals to maintain this crunch like position. The balls are placed on the lower back and are rolled up and down the spine from the crest of the hip to below the scapula with the aid from the legs. The arms do not aid in this rolling movement but aid the abdominals contracting. Perform this 10 to 50 times. This really stretches the lower back while developing the abdominal muscle.

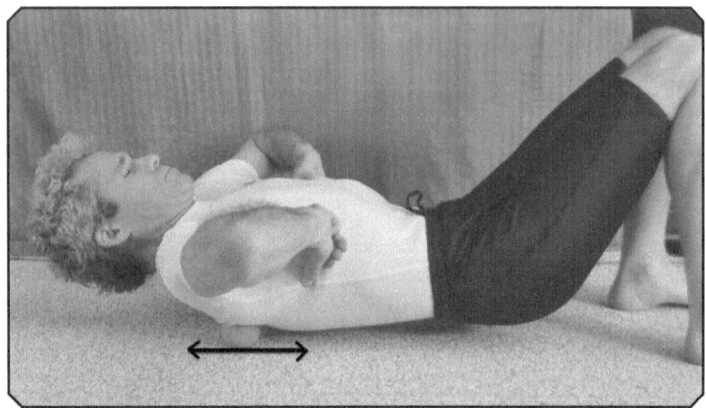

8   Massage the upper back in the chicken wing position with 2 balls.
    Lying on the floor, knees bent and feet close to the butt, arms are
    place in what I like to call the chicken wing position. The elbows
    are at around 90 degrees and off the floor; the hands are on the
    sides somewhere below the armpit. The goal is to spread the scapulas
    apart crating a larger area between the two. This position exposes
    more muscles around the scapula and places other muscle under
    a slight stretch. This aids the effects of the massage. The balls are
    placed on the upper back and rolled up and down with aid from
    the legs One smooth movement up and then down. Keep the balls
    parallel and in sync. Adjust the balls as often as needed. Stay away
    from the spine and scapula. 10 to 50 times.

9   Massage the trapezius (top of shoulders) muscles with 2 balls. Repeat
    exercise 4.

---

10  <u>Massage the neck and scalp with 1 ball.</u> Repeat exercise 5.

---

11  <u>Massage the gluteus and sacral area with 1 ball.</u> This is the same as exercise 1 but with one ball. This allows slight roll to the side and massage more of the gluteus muscles. Do the right side first then left.

---

12  <u>Massage the lower back with 1 ball. Right side first, then left side left side.</u> This is the same as exercise 2 but with one ball. This allows for a deeper massage with more pressure focused on one ball. Right side first.

---

13  <u>Massage the upper back and shoulder area with 1 ball, right side first, then the left side.</u> This is the same as exercise 3 but with one ball. Right side first.

---

14  <u>Massage the trapezius muscle with one ball; right side first then left side.</u> This is the same as exercise 4 but with one ball. Right side first.

---

15  <u>Massage neck and scalp with 1 ball, right side first then left side.</u> Repeat exercise 5.

---

16 <u>Massage the gluteus and sacral area with 1 ball.</u> This is the same as exercise 1 but with one ball.

------------------------------------------------------------

17 <u>zigzag patterns up and down each side of the back. 1 ball.</u> The body is in the same position as exercise 7, the crunch position. With this exercise you perform zigzag patterns up and down the entire length of the back form the crest of the hips to the top of the shoulders. Zigzag every couple of inches completing any where from 10 to 20 zigzags each time you go up and down the back. Go up and down the back 2 to 10 times, Right side first. Strum those muscles like a guitar string. Stay on areas that are tight or sore if you desire. This is about what the pattern would like. Be careful not to let the ball roll over the vertebrae, hips and shoulder blades.

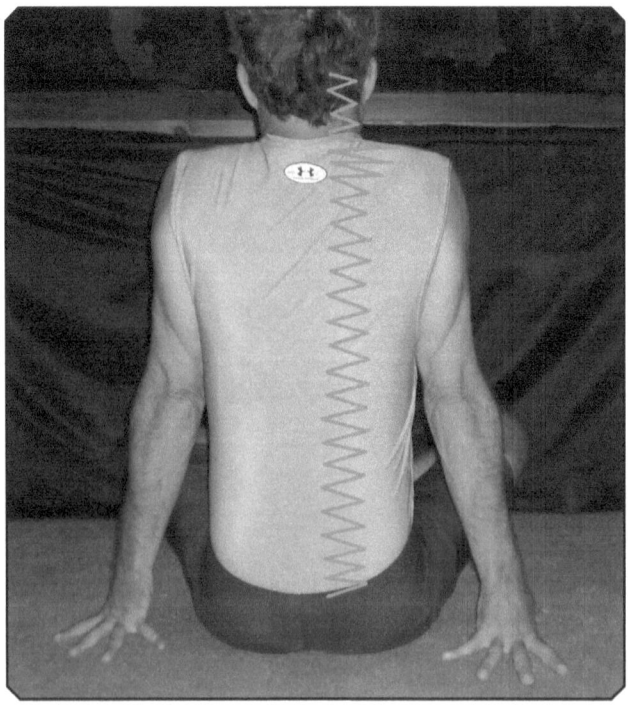

18  <u>Massage the trapezius muscle with one ball</u>. This is the same as exercise 4 but with one ball. Right side first then left side.

---

19  <u>Massage neck and scalp with 1 ball, right side first then left side,</u> This is the same as exercise 5 but with one ball. Right side first.

---

20  <u>Massage the lower back (in the crunch position) with 1 ball. Right side first, then left side left side</u>. This is the same as exercise 7 but with one ball. Right side first.

---

21  <u>Massage the upper back (in the chicken wing position) and shoulder area with 1 ball.</u> This is the same as exercise 8 but with one ball. Right side first

---

22  <u>Massage the trapezius muscle with one ball</u>. This is the same as exercise 4 but with one ball. Right side first then left side.

---

23  <u>Massage neck and scalp with 1 ball,</u> Repeat exercise 5

---

## CONTRAINDICATIONS

Contraindication means that it may not be advisable to massage yourself performing the ripper or even the couch potato. I caution you, when in doubt, always refer to a doctor. DO YOUR BODY NO HARM. Here's the list of when not to give yourself or receive a massage.

1. Massage, especially deep pressure, will make a cold or flu worse. A fever is definitely a no go situation.
2. Any acute inflammation like arthritis, neuritis, or dermatitis. Be cautious to stay away from those areas, if a massage is given at all.
3. Any inflammation from tissue damage. Stay off the discolored, swollen areas.
4. Any visible bacteria infections, (pus)
5. Osteoporosis (bone deterioration) or any frail, old people
6. Anywhere there are varicose veins
7. Swollen, painful veins known as phlebitis or any kind of circulatory abnormality
8. High blood pressure is not for the ripper, but maybe the couch potato. If done lightly, massage will aid in lowering of blood pressure
9. If you are extremely tired or fatigued
10. Any kind of skin problem
11. Scoliosis (crooked spine). Massage must be given with extreme care. Gravity Yoga will help this condition.
12. Any kind of disease or condition see you doctor.

# CHAPTER 5

# AEROBIC FITNESS

It is well established that regular aerobic exercise also know as "cardio" will help you live a healthier, happier life. If performed correctly, it greatly reduces the risk of sickness and injury. Most importantly, Cardio forces blood and nutrients into the tissues. Most studies have shown that 20 minutes, 3 times a week is the minimum amount to achieve good aerobic fitness. That's all!

Aerobic fitness is usually considered low intensity. And can take many forms. Walking briskly is considered one of the safest and most convenient form of cardio, if you can get your heart rate to the desired level. There have been many studies to show which forms of aerobic exercises are the best. The elliptical machine seems to be better than the treadmill or the bike for many reasons. Elliptical machines are safer because they are low impact. Elliptical machines also involve exercising the arms as well as the legs. Treadmills and bicycles don't utilize the arms. The cross-country ski machines work well but it's still not as good as an elliptical machine. An elliptical machine requires the arms to push and pull against a resistance, whereas cross-country ski machines, you are just pulling with your arms. With aerobic, the more muscles being used, the better the training effect. Swimming is very low impact, but it's not easily accessible. Some people consider swimming as the best cardio exercise. Take everything very slow at first; many people have heart attacks on the treadmill. Of coarse, always consult with your doctor before starting any kind of exercise or diet.

For aerobic exercise to yield healthy results the heart should be beating at 50% to 80% of your maximum heart rate. The goal is to reach 70% to 80% of your maximum heart rate for 20 minutes.

Your maximum heart rate is determined by the simple formula, **220 – your age= maximum heart rate**. So if you were 40 years old your formula would be 220-40=180. 180 beats per minute is your max heart rate for a 40-year-old person. Now to find your ideal aerobic heart rate multiply 180 x .50 = 90. Now multiply 180 x .80 = 144. So for a 40-year-old person your heart rate should be between 90 and 144 beats per minute, sustained for 20 minutes 3 times a week. 70% to 80% gives the best cardiovascular results.

Now if you are doing aerobic exercise to lose body fat, there are studies that show lower intensity workouts burn increased amounts of fat than do the higher intensity workouts. Somewhere around 50% to 60% of maximum heart rate burn more fat than at the higher rates of 70% to 80%. The higher rates give the best results cardiovascular conditioning. It's kind of a trade off.

If nothing else, do aerobics for the rush! Cardio releases endorphins, which are like natural heroin without the side effects. It's a natural painkiller. However here are some other good reasons for performing aerobics.

1.  It increases stamina and reduces fatigue
2.  Studies have proven people that are aerobically fit live longer.
3.  It activates your immune system, keeping you disease free.
4.  Keeps your muscles toned and strong so you may enjoy life
5.  It keeps your mind intact as we age.
6.  It lowers cholesterol and raises HDL (good fat)

7. It can help to eliminate heart disease, diabetes, obesity, stroke, high blood pressure, some cancers and osteoporosis.
8. Improves blood flow to all parts of the body.
9. Makes you happy and relaxed. Probable the endorphins.
10. Strengthens the heart and keeps your arteries clear.

I would like to add that even though studies have shown that people are aerobically fit could live longer; there is evidence that you can do too much aerobics. Anything that speeds up your metabolism has the potential to take years off your life. This is contrary to what many people believe in that a faster metabolism can keep you thin and therefore can make you live longer. This is not so true. It is known that people with slow metabolism can live the longest, but only if they are thin. The only way people with slow metabolism can be thin is to have a proper diet consisting of lots of vegetables and maybe lean meats, or not eat much. People with slow metabolism that don't eat a proper diet gain weight quickly and have higher illness and death rates, What I'm trying to say is, A slow metabolism has the potential for the longest lifespan but only if one is thin. So I recommend only doing the bare minimum of 20 minutes a day, 3 times a week for an aerobic workout. It is better to keep your metabolism slow and eat correctly then to have a fast metabolism and eat correctly. Now if you are training for sport, of coarse you may want to customize your aerobic workout for that particular sport. If you are a soccer player, of coarse you will have a need to run as the main portion of an aerobic workout.

Steroids put your metabolism into overdrive. Like I mentioned before, people with slow metabolisms have the potential to live the longest. Steroids increase the metabolism. If you want to die young, do the steroids.

Staying hydrated during aerobic exercise is vital. Water is quickly loss through sweat and respiration and if not replaced it can cause anything from headaches to cramps to even death. Large amounts of waste are produced during prolong exercise and water flushes the wastes out of the cells. Water also brings the nutrients required for prolonged exercise. Water also cools the body with sweat as well as maintain your blood pressure. Drink plenty of water even if it means going to the bathroom often. It is advised that you should drink water before during and after any prolonged exercise. It is recommended that you allow your body to cool down and return to normal before you hydrate after an event. The amount of water needed depends on many factors like climate, duration of exercise and initial hydration levels. Your urine should be clear and odorless if you are hydrated properly. That's probable the easiest way to know if you are properly hydrated.

Of coarse if you are elderly or haven't worked out in some time, take it slow. Always get your doctors approval before starting any fitness program.

# Chapter 6

# NUTRITION

This section of the book is based on current nutritional science. This is what is being taught in colleges and Universities. The core of this book is exercise. However, nutrition is vastly important to general health and well-being. You can exercise all you want, but if you don't eat properly, you are doing little to improve yourself. It is my duty to explain what I know about nutrition. I would not being doing you any favors if I with held any information that might keep you from being as healthy as possible. Most illnesses are self-induced because of a bad diet. Therefore illness can be reversed or reduced through aggressive nutritional diets.

Let me start out saying, foods like milk, soda, margarine, white bread, sugar, and pasteurized American cheese are not healthy foods. My goal as concerning nutrition is too summarize what I have learned from textbooks, journals and reputable authors. My specialty is fitness and innovations in exercise. The fitness sections of the book are all from my own discoveries derived from experiences and my gift in understanding bio- mechanics. I can tell you what you should or shouldn't eat, but I'm not a chef. I can only give you the basics. For books with great recipes I suggest Dr Joel Furhman and Dr Gary Null. Both have tasty recipes and explain nutrition in great depth.

Nutrition could be the most important of topics when it comes to America's problem with obesity. Obesity is the largest predictor of one's health and quality of living. However optimal health and weight loss can only be obtained from eating large amounts of nutrient rich food and exercise. Nutrients are vitamins, minerals, fibers and micronutrients. Micronutrients are all those helpful chemical compounds found in foods. Fruits and vegetables, particularly green leafy vegetables are high in micronutrients. Mushrooms. Berries, onions and green vegetables are all high in micronutrients and low calorie. Micronutrients reduce hunger, make you feel great and fight cancer. Meat, potatoes and bread have no micronutrients. It's not natural to have heart disease and high blood pressure, as you get older. Your health is the greatest gift you can give your body.

Leafy- greens such as kale, Swiss chard, collards and spinach are the most nutrient dense foods. Some fruits like blueberries are high in anthocyanins, which are anti-aging. A tomato contains more than 10,000 micronutrients. Compounds found in cabbage sprouts and broccoli (cruciferous vegetables) removes toxins in our cells and helps prevent cancer. Peppers, beats and tomatoes fight cancerous changes in cells. Oranges and apples, protect us from heart disease. You won't ever be able to put thousands of these micronutrients into one pill. And many of these helpful compounds haven't even been discovered yet. Foods that lack nutrients are called empty calories and should be avoided. I suggest eating 2 large salads a day. A green salad is less than 100 calories. And can weigh a pound or more. By the way, salad means raw and uncooked.

If you don't have the time to consume that much salad, there is the juice diet alternative. It's a great idea to convert fresh vegetable and fruit into a juice. There are many delicious recipes and it is very convenient. I am in no way indorsing the fruit juice that you buy at the store that is bad in so many ways. I'm talking about the juice that is made at home from fresh vegetables and fruits. However, there is evidence that chewing your food is the best way to absorb the nutrients, and that processing food in a blender oxidizes the nutrients, rendering them ineffective.

Don't be a gluten glutton. Gluten is a protein found mainly in wheat. Food manufacturers add gluten to foods for many reasons but mainly to glue their product together and keep it from falling apart. There's lots of gluten in processed foods, MSG, modified cornstarch. Many people have allergies to gluten called celiac disease. Even if you don't have this allergy, gluten is very bad for your health. Gluten coats your intestines and prevents the absorption of nutrients. Gluten is linked to cancer and many illnesses and can even alter DNA.

Dairy is anything but healthy for you. First of all dairy has a strong association with prostate cancer. It also has high fat content and most contain added hormones and antibiotics. These hormones cause cancer and the antibiotics create havoc to the immune system. You certainly don't want to be eating that. Our government has dairy as a building block for its food pyramid. What a joke. The pyramid also has bread, cereal rice and pasta in this pyramid, which is highly disputed by most nutritionist. Our Government is telling you the wrong things to eat.

Dairy and meat protein (excluding fish) cause inflammation. All cancers are cause by inflammation. If you can't eliminate dairy and meat, then only one serving every day or two will be enough. If red meat is eliminated from your diet, be careful to get protein and iron from other sources. Fish contain Omega 3 fatty acids, which are anti-inflammatory. Wild caught fish is the best. Mushrooms are a great anti-inflammatory making it an outstanding cancer fighting food. Foods high in folic acid like green vegetables are anti inflammatory. Papaya and pineapple have a chemical compound that reduces inflammation,

Staying hydrated is of extreme importance. Of coarse if you are eating plenty of fresh vegetables and fruits you may need less water because of the large water content fruits and veggies have. Water is needed for every system in your body. It is key for removing toxins and temperature control. Your urines should be clear and odorless, if not you aren't getting enough water.

Obesity is a combination of bad food choices, inactivity and genetics. Studies have shown that physically inactivity is the strongest environmental determinant of total body and central abdominal fat mass. Studies have shown that abdominal fat is the best predictor of health. Proper nutrition and exercise is the secret to prevent and cure illnesses. First year medical students learn that all medications are toxic. So why medicated yourself? You have every thing you need to be healthy, by eating and exercising correctly. It is a well-established fact that thin people live a much longer and healthier life. Monkey's that were fed a calorie-restricted diets lived 30%longer. The thinner the better! Not including anorexia, of coarse.

There are three sources of fuel that your body burns for fuel, Carbohydrates, fats and proteins.

**Protein**. Proteins could be the most important of the three fuel sources, (proteins, carbohydrates and fats). They are required for every chemical reaction that takes place in our muscles and tissues. Proteins are the basis for how our bodies move, functions and regenerate. The body cannot store protein, unlike carbohydrates and fats. Therefore, if you are not consuming protein through out the day, your body will actually start taking protein from muscles and organs to replace those being expended by bodily processes. You will actually start digesting your intestines first, which is normal. It's your body's way of regulating protein levels. If protein is not being consumed then your muscle tissue is next to be used. In a sense you are eating yourself in a process called "muscle cannibalism". That's one reason old people look frail. They ate themselves! However, if you eat too much animal and milk protein can harm your kidneys and lungs. An excessive amount of animal and milk protein raises insulin-like growth factors, which are, linked to high rates of breast and prostate cancer. Most dairy and meat products have added hormones and antibiotics, which can only lead to you getting fat and sick. In general, it can be a fine balancing act to get the correct amount of protein. Proteins from plant sources are highly desirable. Americans eat way too much protein and red meat. You need just under 60 grams of protein a day,(more if you're an athlete), which isn't a lot, but is best to be consumed throughout the day. However if you eat a lot of leafy green vegetables you can eat less often. This is because high fiber, high micronutrient, vegetables slow down absorption of nutrients into the blood stream. 100 calories of broccoli has more protein then 100 calories of sirloin steak. The old school of thought that animal protein is more complete or better than vegetable protein has been determined to be false. It is best to get your protein from plant based sources. If you are an athlete or very active you may consider taking a plant based protein supplement.

Inflammation occurs when eating the wrong foods. All cancers are cause by inflammation so it's a good idea to stay away from these foods. Animal and milk protein cause inflammation so it's a good idea to stay away from theses foods, or al least limit them to one serving every day or two. If you eliminate red meat from your diet, be careful to get enough iron in you diet from other sources. There are vegetable based protein powders on the market that will help replace missing protein if you don't want to eat dairy or meat. Fish however are anti-inflammatory. Fish, have Omega 3 fatty acids that reduce inflammation and are a good source of protein.

There are two basic schools of thought here. The first is that eating often, 5-6 times a day, is healthy because it creates an even flow of protein and sugar into the bloodstream. This even flow of protein is important because the body does not store protein. Without this continuous flow of protein in the bloodstream, your body will start to extract protein from the muscles and organs. In a sense you are eating yourself, which is, counter productive to muscle growth and general health. The other school of thought is that eating 1-2 meals a day or even fasting for a day, your Allows the body to detoxify. There are also studies that show that the brain can actually improve from fasting. But you must eat lots of fresh vegetables and fruit. Studies have shown that eating less frequently correlates to a longer life span even when the same amounts of calories are consumed. And fasting has been found to increase neuron growth in the brain. If you are only going to eat 1 or 2 meals a day, they should consist of lots of green leafy vegetables and other complex carbohydrates as to avoid blood sugar spikes. Eating three, nutritious meals a day seem maybe a way to compromise on these two competing theories.

As you get older, you start loosing muscle faster than you can add from diet alone. Exercise can prevent this. The lost of this muscle mass will increase the aging process and lead to all other kinds of disorders like fat gain, diabetes and Osteoporosis. Your body can produce 10 of the 20 amino acids that are needed to form a protein. So getting these in your diet are paramount. Protein is found in most food. The old way of think is that good sources of protein are meat, fish, seeds, nuts, free-range eggs, milk, cheese and yogurt. I suggest fresh caught wild salmon. However I strongly suggest that all milk and fatty meats be avoided. However, all of your protein needs can be met if you eat enough fruits and vegetables, but that means 2 pounds of veggies. That's about 2 shoeboxes worth of veggies. We Americans get way to much protein and too much protein can be linked to almost every disease. Lots of green leafy vegetables and small amounts of lean meats have plenty of protein. A banana has as much protein as mother's milk. The body requires somewhere around 45 to 90 grams of protein. Everyone is different. Athletes' may require up to twice that amount of protein to allow for growth, repair and recovery of muscle. Once you lose muscle, it can be very difficult to get back what you have lost. Some suggest taking whey (milk protein) as a supplement, before and after workouts. But once again, you don't want too much milk protein because of its links with many aliments. You don't want to risk all the side effects if possible. I suggest vegetable base protein powder, if you require more protein. Remember it's a fine balancing act between too much protein and not enough. And many top nutritionists believe fruits and vegetables, with very little milk and animal protein, in your diet should meet all your protein needs. That means lots of raw veggies, fruits and some nuts. If you are an athlete you have to consume more protein. This can be impractical for many.

**Carbohydrates**. Carbohydrates are the body's first and primary source of energy. They provide fuel for every bodily process such as the immune system, nervous system, cardiovascular system, blood clotting and growth. Foods rich in carbohydrates when eaten in their natural state, are lower in calories and higher in fiber, than fatty foods, processed foods, or animal products.

There are basically 2 types of carbohydrates, simple and complex.

Simple carbohydrates (sugars) are quickly digested and rapidly converted into energy. They are often used as energy boosters during exercise, however this energy is not sustainable over long periods of time. Frequent large intakes of simple carbohydrates can lead to havoc on your blood sugar count. Large increases followed by sharp decreases in blood sugar can create a condition called hypoglycemia or diabetes mellitus. These sugars are why food taste sweet. Many top nutritionists equate sugar to poison and should be avoided. Refined carbohydrates, sweets, wheat flower and some fruit juices can enter the bloodstream to quickly, raising your triglycerides and increase your rate of a heart attack. Pasta is not healthy, Its poison!

Complex carbohydrates (starch, fiber and glycogen) are long chains of simple sugars linked together by a hydrogen atom. Because of their size they are released into the bloodstream at a much slower and steadier rate, than simple sugars. This makes them highly desirable. Complex carbohydrates will not make blood sugar levels fluctuate therefore it's not necessary to eat them may times a day.

Starch, fiber and glycogen are complex carbohydrates. Starches are found in potatoes and rice. Fiber is found in whole grains, vegetables, legumes, fruit skins and potatoes skins. Make sure that all skins are washed to avoid pesticides. Organic produce is pesticide free. GMO's or produce that has been changed genetically has been linked to many diseases. Why the USA allows them is beyond me. Most of the world has them banned or at least has it labeled on food. Here in the USA we don't label GMO's. We are the only industrialized country that allows this to happen?

Fiber cannot be broken down into sugars like starches and glycogen. Fiber removes waste and toxins and increases the effectiveness of the digestion process. Fiber is extremely important to the digestive system. Of coarse fresh fruits and veggies are the highest in fiber. The typical American diet is dangerously lacking fiber. This leads to many problems like constipation, varicose veins, diabetes and cancer. There is evidence that just sprinkling Metamucil on French fries or eating a high fiber candy bar, does not get the same results as eating fruits and vegetables. 50 to 100 grams of fiber form fresh fruit and vegetables is desirable. Refined grains like pasta and white bread and white rice have had their fiber removed and have little to no nutritional value. They are even declared as poison by some top nutritionist.

Glycogen is the third type of complex carbohydrate. Ingested glycogen comes from meat and can only be stored minimally so you need to consume additional complex carbohydrates to replenish, those being used. If not, exhaustion sets in.

It is advised that large quantities of complex carbohydrates are consumed for athletes 3 hours before exercise. A general rule for everyone is a ratio of 45:35:20 where as carbohydrates are 45% of your diet, protein is 35% and fats are 20%. However, with a diet of fresh fruits and veggies and little to no lean meat, you never have to worry about proportions. You can never eat too much on this kind of diet. You can eat all you want of fresh fruit and vegetables, if limit your meat to 3 servings a week. Salad dressing and oil is not good for you. Limit that to one tablespoon a day. Flaxseed oil is by far the best of all the oils and is desirable. This is the best diet. Nuts are good for you even though high in oil and fat. However these are highly nutritious. If pistachios or walnuts are consumed before a meal, they will increase the body's ability to absorb vastly more of the nutrition form other foods. If you are overweight, no more than a handful of uncooked nuts are advised. Cooking changes good fat into bad fat. Avoid large portions of carbohydrates before bed because this can become fat. If you eat plenty of vegetables and only a small amount of lean meat (2-3 times a week), you never have to worry about fat.

There is a tool that measures how carbohydrates are ranked. It is call, 'The Glycemic index. This is very important in the prevention and control of diabetes. Foods are ranked in the amount of glucose in the blood, two hours after consumption. This is a measurement to minimize insulin related conditions like diabetes. In a general rule, it is more desirable to chose food low on the glycemic index to prevent blood sugar and insulin spikes. Complex carbohydrates are ranked low and simple carbohydrates are ranked high in the glycemic index. Strawberries, one of my favorites, are low on the glycemic index.

**Fats**. (Triglycerides, phospholipids and sterols) They are essential to your diet. All your fat needs, can be met, by eating green leafy vegetables. The body will convert food fat to body fat easily and quickly. Olive oil and other cooking and salad oils are not healthy nor are they good for weight loss. Oils lose their nutritional value once there are removed from the source. Bottom line, fats are oil and will add to your waistline, which will lead to many types of illness. As a result, diets like The Mediterranean Diet that replaces "bad fats with good fats" are only good if you are close to your ideal body weight. The Mediterranean Diet also suggests eating pasta and Italian bread. This will make losing weight difficult, and has links to cancer. If you are thin and get lots of exercise that a tablespoon of olive oil is not going to hurt, but for the vast majority of overweight Americans, no oil is best. Healthy fats that come from nuts, seeds and avocadoes should be limited to small amount, if your goal is losing weight. Olive oil has none of the phytonutrients that olives have. However, all extracted fat causes cancer because they are empty calories with no nutritional value. This causes not only cancer but also obesity and premature aging.

Triglycerides are the most common fat and responsible for many of structural functions of the body.

Phospholipids and are fats manufactured by the body and essential for proper bodily functions. The third class is sterols such as cholesterol.

Cholesterol is a sterol type fat needed for proper health and functioning of your body. Although in large numbers cholesterol is bad, it is however, essential for every bodily function. LDL or low-density lipoproteins cholesterol are the bad cholesterols. These clog arteries and cause heart disease. The higher your LDL level the greater chance of heart disease. HDL or high-density lipoproteins are the good cholesterols. HDL lowers the levels of LDL in the bloodstream and tissues. HDL reverses the bad effects of LDL

Fats are required for many functions of the body such as the absorption of vitamins. A, D, K AND E. Fats are required for proper development of cells. They also protect and insulate the organs. Fats are fuel for strenuous and endurance activities.

Excess fatty acids that are not used become stored as fat in adipose tissue, muscles or liver. Only the fat stored in muscle is used for energy purposes.

Triglycerides are the most common class of lipid or fat and there are two types, saturated and non-saturated. Non-saturated is liquid at room temp and is considered the healthy one of the two. Saturated fat is harmful to your health. Where as non-saturated fat is healthy, and only becomes harmful when heat is applied, hydrating it. I other words, cooking even good fat is bad for you. Coconut oil maybe the exception to this rule.

The body requires two essential fatty acids, linoleic and alpha-linoleic acid. These must be met in your diet and should be 10 to 20 % of your macronutrient intake. Diets that maintain this healthy ratio help the body not to store fat. They reduce heart disease and stroke. Essential fatty acids are required for proper nerve and brain functions. Once again, eating lots of fresh vegetables and fruits gives you all the correct amounts of fats.

Omega-3s are derived from essential fatty acids. They come from eating cold-water fish like salmon, trout, tuna, cod, and mackerel. Omega 3's can also come from a vegetable sources. Microalgae is now producing omega 3's in a capsule form. This is highly desirable. Omega 3's increase strength and aerobic capabilities, in addition to lowering cholesterol. Most Americans don't eat enough omega 3's but eat too much omega 6. Omega 6 promotes inflammation whereas omega 3 is anti-inflammatory. Inflammation causes disease. Omega 6 is found in meat.

Saturated fats and Trans-fatty acids cause heart disease, diabetes, clogged arteries and high cholesterol. Hydrogenated trans fat are no better for you than saturated fats. These can be found in dairy and meats and artificially in processed foods. They increase the shelf life of food but are terrible for you. The daily allowances for these fats are 1% of your total diet. I suggest O% or none. There is possible one exception to this rule and its coconut oil. Although it is saturated fat, it is not know to have any side effects. In fact, it is advise to cook with coconut oil, if you have to cook with oil. All other oils, even the healthy fats become saturated at high temperatures. Saturation causes heart disease, clogged arteries, diabetes, etc.

Sources of fat:

* Mono-unsaturated fats are from olives, avocadoes, canola oils and peanut oil.

* Poly-unsaturated fats are from corn oil, safflower oil and sesame oil.
* Omega-3 fatty acids are from cod, salmon, sardines trout and mackerel and many plant sources.
* Trans fats are from fried foods, pizza dough, packaged snack foods, microwave Popcorn, margarine, cookies, and crackers
* Saturated fats come from whole milk, butter, cream, cheeses, lard and ice cream.
* Cholesterol comes from meats, dairy, egg yolks, poultry, fish and eggs. The body also produces it. And is not needed in our diet

It is recommended for healthy individuals to eat no more than 30% of fat and less than 10% of saturated fats. Many nutritionist say no saturated fat at all. For weight loss it is recommend that only 20% of your diet should come from fat. Less than 15% fat is bad for your bodily functions. A reduced fat diet is better than just reducing overall calories diets. Essential fats should be 1 to 2% of daily caloric intake. Once again, eating plenty of leafy green vegetables and small amounts of lean meat is the best diet and you never have to worry about eating too much or proper proportions.

**Vitamins,**

Vitamins play an important role in the proper functioning of metabolic processes within our bodies. The also provide many health benefits and can improve athletic performance. Most vitamins are needed in our diets because our bodies can't produce them. If a vitamin is missing from our diet, metabolic activity is impaired. Although vitamins have nutritional content, they are not metabolized for energy. They do assist in energy production. There are many vitamins in the form of micronutrients that are not yet discovered. Eating plenty of fresh fruits and veggies is paramount because no pill or supplement can ever replace a compound that has not yet been discovered.

Though it is not necessary to know all the vitamins and minerals to live a healthy life, I thought it's interesting and you might want to learn about it. After all, if you eat a proper diet you will get all the nutrition that you need.

There are 2 basic types of vitamins, water soluble (B complex and C), and fat- soluble (A, D, E and K). Fat-soluble can be stored in the liver and you can overdose on them. Water-soluble vitamins can only be store briefly so they must be consumed daily. And there is no chance of overdosing on them, however much is lost in food preparation. Eating raw fresh vegetables has the most nutrition. As soon as heat is applied to them or are processed in any way, vitamins lose their nutritional value. It's best to eat vitamins directly from their source. If you need vitamin C, eat an orange and not a pill.

I've decided to list the conventional vitamins. I want to stress that many vitamins in the form of phytochemicals (micronutrients) are not yet described or even discovered by science. No one knows how important these micronutrients are. are. Once again, if you eat a diet rich in green leafy veggies and a little lean meat you never have to worry about what you maybe lacking in your diet. I fact, if you eat a proper diet, then you really don't have to concern yourself with all these vitamins and minerals that I have listed. You may find it interesting though and knowledge is power.

Just because I listed things like milk as sources of a particular vitamin does not mean that I am personally indorsing milk.

Water-soluble vitamins

- B complex plays a crucial role in the metabolism of fats, carbohydrates and protein

- B-1 main function is to aid in carbohydrate function and plays a role in appetite Stimulation. It's found in pork, rice bran, oatmeal, potatoes and asparagus.
- B-2 plays a major roll in the production of energy and cellular respiration. Its found in Fish, eggs, poultry, milk, yogurt, nuts and green vegetables.
- B-3 is needed in the production of energy, protein synthesis and the synthesis of hormones and amino acids.
- B-5 has a key role in the synthesis and metabolism of fatty acids. It is found in whole grains, liver, legumes, meats and eggs.
- B-6 it functions in the break down of proteins and the metabolism of amino acids and fats. It is found in liver, meats, whole grains, nuts, bananas, soybeans and rice.
- B-7 is produce in the intestines so deficiencies are rare. It is require for amino acid and fatty acids. It also promotes healthy bone marrow, nerve tissue, hair and skin. Its main source is egg yolk, milk, liver,
- B-9 is required for the synthesis of DNA and RNA. It metabolizes amino acids. It is also needed for the production of red blood cells, tissue and muscle growth. It Comes from dark green leafy vegetables, red meat, salmon and liver.
- B-12 is needed for proper brain function and nervous system. It helps in many metabolic functions and is often referred to as the "energy vitamin. Main sources are shellfish, liver, eggs, milk, lamb and poultry.

Vitamin C. This is an antioxidant that can be produced by the body. It is important for protein production and plays an important role in maintaining healthy tissues and cells. It plays a major role in fighting infection and promoting overall health. Main food sources are citrus fruits, tomatoes, broccoli, strawberries, peppers, spinach and potatoes.

Fat-soluble vitamins. As mentioned before, these can become toxic if too much are taken. However many people that are on low fat diets are at risk for deficiencies. Because these vitamins are fat soluble, fat, in one's diet is required for the absorption of these vitamins. Eating fresh fruits and veggies will supply everything you need in the proper dosages.

Vitamin A is for vision, cellular growth, bone development, and a healthy immune and reproductive system. It is found in egg yolks, milk, fish, carrots, cantaloupe broccoli and leafy green vegetables. It is now recommended that people do not take supplements of vitamin A, isolate beta –carotene or folic acid.

Vitamin D aids in hormonal activity and performs as a signaling mechanism in bone and cell growth. In the presence of sunlight, the body manufactures vitamin D. It's main function is in the development of bones and teeth. A lack of vitamin D leads to bad teeth and brittle bones. Vitamin D is found in cod liver oil, fish eggs, butter, cream and milk. However I do not agree with eating, butter, cream and most dairy products.

Vitamin E is an antioxidant and its main function is the formation of red blood cells. Being an antioxidant vitamin E aids in minimizing cellular damage. It helps to synthesize RNA and DNA. Vitamin E is necessary for the reproductive system and is also important for athletic performance. Sources of Vitamin E are wheat germ oil, nuts, liver and leafy green vegetables.

Vitamin K breaks down in the presence of sunlight. The main function of vitamin K is blood clotting. Vitamin K produces prothrombin, and a deficiency of this will cause hemorrhaging.

## MINERALS

Dietary minerals are essential to every living organism. Minerals come from the water and earth and are absorbed by plants and animals. Minerals are essential for synthesizing of hormones, building of bones, contracting the muscles, regulating the heart, conductivity of neurons and vital for a healthy immune system.

There are two types of Mineral: macro-minerals and trace minerals. Macro- minerals are, calcium, phosphorous, magnesium, sodium, chloride, potassium and sulfur. These are required in large quantities in order to have healthy bodily functions. The trace minerals are, boron, chromium, copper, fluoride, iron, iodine, manganese, selenium, vanadium and zinc. These are required in small amounts but the body is dependant on all minerals for proper health.

Macro- Minerals. These are usually digested in large quantities with dosages exceeding 100 milligrams a day. The excretion of minerals is through bodily fluids like sweat and urine. Some macro- nutrients are also referred to electrolytes. These help regulate water flow between blood vessels and cells.

<u>Calcium</u> is requited for healthy bones, teeth and gums. It is need for proper heart and nervous system functions. Calcium is necessary for blood clotting and helps stabilize bodily functions. It is found in cheese, milk, yogurt, kale, shellfish, salmon and broccoli. I do not suggest any dairy products. There is just to many problems associated with it.

<u>Magnesium</u> is important for structural and metabolic functions in the body. It assists in the formation of, teeth, muscles, bones, tissues and nerves. Magnesium aids in absorption of calcium and potassium. It is also required to relax muscles. It also develops cardiac tissue and regulates blood pressure. It is found in whole grains, nut, legumes, green leafy vegetables and fruits.

<u>Phosphorous</u> is required in the formation of bone, teeth and the formation of cellular membranes. It is required for the metabolism of fats and carbohydrates. It is essential in cardiac muscle control and cardiac muscle control.

ELECTROLYTES are macro- nutrients that are electrically charged (ions). They are responsible for the flow of water between the cells and the bloodstream. The primary electrolytes are sodium, potassium and chloride.

Chloride is needed for fluid loss and retention as well as the body's acid-base balance. It aids in the formation of hydrochloric acid in the stomach that is required for digestion. Chloride's main source is table salt. It also found in celery, tomatoes, olives Seaweed and processed foods.

Potassium is an electrolyte responsible for all cellular activity, muscle control, cardiac tissue control, nerve transmission and kidney functions. It is found in oranges, bananas, meat, dairy product, poultry and potato skins.

Sodium is an electrolyte responsible for all cellular activity. It helps the body support healthy fluid levels. It is vital for muscle and cardiac contraction and nerve transmission. Sodium aids in the production of hydrochloric acid for the digestive system. It is mainly found in table salt, sports drinks, cheese, ham, smoked meats, processed meats and canned soup. Oh coarse sodium is associated with heart disease and many other health risks.

Sulfur is an acid- forming mineral that purifies the blood, helps fight bacteria and protects cellular protoplasm. It helps to stimulate the liver to create bile and protect the body against toxins like radioactive elements and pollutants. It is found in Brussels sprouts, cabbage, dried beans kale, eggs, soybeans, onions, meats, wheat germ and turnips.

TRACE MINERALS.

The trace minerals are, boron, chromium, copper, fluoride, iron, iodine, manganese, selenium, vanadium and zinc. These are needed in smaller amounts than Macro- nutrients, Many Trace minerals act as enzymes that activate other molecules. They are important for activating metabolic functions. Minerals can combine with amino acids to form lager molecules. Warning that one should take care and not take excessive dosages of trace minerals. This can have negative side effects.

Boron is needed for the proper formation of bones and cells. It also aids in the regulation of calcium, magnesium and phosphorous. Boron helps the brain and memory, and reduces arthritis. It is mainly found in green leafy vegetables, fruits nuts, legumes, apples, pears, grains, carrots and broccoli.

Chromium is important for metabolizing fats and carbohydrates. It assists insulin in lowering blood sugar levels. It may also be very important in muscle building. It is found in meat, whole grains, bread, brewer's yeast, brown rice and potatoes.

Copper is needed in the formation of red blood cells. It helps metabolize carbohydrates and fats. Copper is also need to form nerve tissue and acts as an antioxidant to boost your immune system. It is found in shellfish, mushrooms, liver, meat, whole grains and potatoes.

Fluoride helps prevent tooth decay and is important in the formation of teeth and bones. It also helps in the prevention of osteoporosis. The main sour is fluorinated drinking water, oats, grains and tea.

Iodine is involved with cell metabolism. Without iodine the thyroid gland can't synthesize the hormones needed energy production, regulation of metabolism, and normal growth. Iodine helps to control cholesterol and stabilize body weight. Its main source is iodized table salt, halibut, cod, oysters, dairy and seaweed.

Iron is important component of hemoglobin, which carries oxygen to the tissues. Iron is found in red meat, liver, fish poultry, legumes, nuts and bread. Women in child baring tears, Low iron can lead to anemia which deprives your cells of oxygen have at greater risk of low iron. New studies are showing that it lowers the risk of cancer in women.

Manganese is important for energy production and in reproduction. Aided by calcium, it is essential for strong bones and connective tissue. Manganese is also need for the synthesis of fat and sex hormones. It is found in Brussels sprouts, nuts, beans, whole grains, corn, bananas, oatmeal and green leafy vegetables.

Molybdenum activates enzyme activity in energy production, nitrogen metabolism and uric acid production. It also helps prevent toxic build-ups of sulfites. It is found in whole grains, nuts, vegetables, milk and cereals and bread.

Selenium is an antioxidant that protects the body from free- radicals. It has anti aging properties and reduces recovery time after exercise. It boosts the immune system and helps reduce arthritic pain, It is found in shellfish, fish, red meats, grains eggs, liver, garlic and chicken.

Vanadium along with insulin plays a role metabolizing glucose. It inhibits cholesterol synthesis, needed in teeth and bones and important for growth and reproduction. It is found in dill, fish, meat, radishes, snap peas, whole grains and vegetable oil.

Zinc is important for cell growth, cell division and cell repair. Zinc is needed for many processes in our body. It helps in the growth and maintenance of muscle tissue. Zinc is also needed for maturation and maintaining healthy skin, hair and nails. It is found in seafood, oysters, herring, liver, meat, eggs, whole wheat bread oats and maple syrup.

## HERBS

Herbs have been around for centuries and are derived from plants that possess healing or medicinal properties. Some of health conditions that herbs have been used to treat are, diabetes, cancer, asthma, heart disease, hypertension, arthritis, shin conditions, sore throat, colds, hair loss, slow the aging process, reduce stress insomnia, increase memory, aid in digestion, and regulate hormone production. Athletes find them valuable for sprains, inflammation, bruising and pain. Herbalists claim they can cure any aliment with out modern medicine. All spices and herbs should be consumed, except for large amounts of salt.

Not only are herbs good for healing, but also they act as vitamins and minerals for good health and maintenance of your body. Some herbs are "adaptogens" because they increase immune responses in your body. Herbs can be taken every day without negative side effects.

Athletes and bodybuilders have used herbs to gain energy, enhance performance, and increase stamina and strength. Some herbs should be avoided because some athletic governing bodies ban them.

It is believed that herbs in their natural state and much more effective and safer that the concentrated forms produced in laboratories. Everyone should be cautious when using herbs. Some may have negative effects when taken with other drugs or herbs. Prolong use of some herbs can also have negative effects. Some are toxic and should not be inhaled or ingested. Rule of thumb, herbs that are bitter are used for medicinal purposes, and herbs that taste pleasant are not toxic.

I want to stress that everyone is different and we all have different chemical make-ups. What works for one person doesn't mean it will work for another. I suggest that you explore all natural remedies, eating a proper diet, and exercise before making the drastic decision of going on pharmaceutical medications. Your doctor should be advised if you are taking an herb for more than 3 months.

The many anatomical parts of a plant (seeds, fruit, roots, stems, leaves flowers and bark) are used for many health and healing benefits. Many roots and bark have fungicidal and bactericidal properties. Herbs can be consumed in supplements, powders, concentrated liquids', teas, extracts and potions. Some external treatments are using herbal and essential oil blends, topical lotions, massage oils, liniments, and body wraps.

Here is a list of some mainstream herbs

Alfalfa was originally cultivated in the Mediterranean region. Sprouts can be eaten in salads, sandwiches or in a juice. Alfalfa helps to support the immune system, help recover and repair tissue and helps alleviate pain.

Aloe is originally from Africa. It's leaves are filled with jell that is made into juices or lotions. Aloe aids the immune system, promotes recover and repair of tissues, slows the aging process, and aids in digestion.

Astragalus is grown in china. Its root is dried and made into extracts or capsules. It can be used in teas and combined with licorice or ginseng to enhance its effectiveness. Astragalus increase energy, promotes tissue repair, enhances the immune system, acts as a diuretic, aids the adrenal gland and aids in digestion.

Barberry. Originally grown on Japan. The berries, bark and root are use to make capsules, teas, tablets, dried herbs and tinctures. It's active ingredient is alkaloid berberine which is also found in golden seal. Barberry helps the immune system and aids in digestion. It helps to promote the recovery and repair of tissues and help to relieve pain.

Bitter orange comes from Africa and Asia. The fruit and peel can be eaten in capsules, tablets and extracts. It is also made into a topical cream. Bitter orange aids the body in fat loss and acts as a good appetite suppressor.

Black Cohosh comes from the eastern and central region of the United States. The rhizomes and roots are made in teas, tablets, capsules and extracts. Black Cohosh benefits the cardiovascular system, reduce stress, relieve pain, and alleviate menstrual pain.

Black Tea was originally from China. The leaves of the Camellia Sinensis plant are made into tea. Black tea aids in digestion and fat loss and also acts as a diuretic. It is also a great source of caffeine, which could be its downfall, in my opinion.

Burdock comes from the eastern and central United States. The roots are used to make stews and soups. And the leaves are rubbed onto the skin for healing and reduced pain. Burdock aids the immune system, promote repair and recovery of tissue and helps eliminate pain. It also helps to stimulate fat los and purify the blood. It is also a remedy for arthritis.

Cayenne. G. Keep it hot! Capsaicin molecule that makes peppers hot shrinks cancerous tumors. It originates in South America and the pepper is made into a powder. It is used in soups, teas, capsules and tablets. Cayenne improves circulation, assists in digestion, and contains thermogenic properties,

Chamomile Comes from Europe and its flowers have been used as medicine for 1000's of years. Chamomile promotes recovery and repair of tissues, acts as a sleep aids and supports the immune system. It also stimulates appetite.

Dandelion comes from Europe. The leaves, roots, and tops are made into tea. Dandelion promotes tissue repair and increase energy levels. It helps gastrointestinal problems. Cleanse the blood and liver, and increase bile production. Dandelion improves organ function and is used as a diuretic.

Evening Primrose comes from all over the United States. Its oil is extracted and made into a capsule. Evening primrose enhances the cardiovascular system, supports the immune system and aids in digestion and helps reduce pain. It also helps with menstrual cramps, eczema and arthritis.

Fenugreek goes back to 1500 BC used by the Egyptian. It can be ingested in capsule form or made into an ointment for the skin. Fenugreek aids in weight loss by suppressing the appetite. It is also used for treating the symptoms of diabetes, stimulating the production of milk, reduce fever, lower cholesterol and lubricate the intestines. Fenugreek is a great laxative.

Flaxseed provides omega 3s which reduces the chance of diabetes, heart disease and cancer. A tablespoon a day is good stuff!

Garcinia (mongosteen). Garcinia kola nut, fruit of mongosteen is grown in Polynesia, Asia, Australia and Africa. It can be eaten. This suppresses the appetite and increases energy levels.

Garlic comes from Central Asia. It can be eaten raw, cooked, dried, or made into capsules or tablets. There is a liquid concentrated form also. Garlic enhances the cardiovascular system and acts to ease stress.

Ginger comes from Asia and the roots can be cooked or eaten raw. It is also dried and made into capsules, tablets and teas. Ginger boosts the immune system, helps to improve the cardiovascular system and relieve nausea and diarrhea. It also stimulates circulation and cleanses the colon.

Ginkgo originates from Asia. The leaves are made into an extract and made into capsules and teas. Ginkgo is know for improving memory, slows down the aging process and helps the cardiovascular system.

Ginseng comes from Asia. It's root is dried and made into capsules, tablets, extracts, topical creams and teas. Ginseng increases energy levels, and promotes tissue repair. It helps to control blood sugar levels, boost the immune system and increase the effectiveness of antibiotics. Ginseng is often used to treat impotence. It increases lung function, stimulates the appetite and normalizes blood pressure.

Gotu Kola comes from the West Indies, Africa, China, Indonesia and Brazil. The plant is dried and made into capsules and tablets. Gotu kola promotes recovery and repair of tissues and increases energy levels. It may also increase concentration and memory function.

Green Tea was originally from China. It helps to maintain high energy levels and aids in weight loss.

Licorice comes from Turkey, Greece and Asia. The root is dried and made into tablets, capsules or an extract. Licorice helps reducing muscle spasm, increase mucus flow through the lungs and bronchial tubes, reduce stress and inflammation and treating colds.

Psyllium comes from the plant Plantago ovato. The seeds and husks are removed and the plant is ingested. It is commonly used as a laxative and aids in fat and weight loss.

Spirulina is blue green algae grown of Mexico and Africa. It aids in weight loss, helps to improve the inflammation caused by allergies and helps to lower blood sugar levels.

White willow bark comes from the Salix Alba tree Europe and North America. The bark is ground up and made into a capsule or topical cream. Chewing on the bark can also release salicin, which is the active ingredient. It acts as a painkiller without side effects and ids in weight loss.

Wu-long tea comes from the plant; Camellia sinensis. The leaves are bruised and dried, then made into a tea. It is used for weight loss because it increases the metabolic rate and fat oxidation.

Yerba Mate is grown in South America, Australia, Spain and Italy. The leaves are dried and made into tea. It plays a role in cell regeneration and increase energy levels.

Yohimbe Bark is dried and ground into a powder. It helps to improve sexual impotence and increase energy levels. It is also used to treat angina and hypertension.

## Heart disease.

Our nations number one killer. A good diet and exercise can insulate you from this disease. There is a strong relationship between eating animal protein and heart disease. It's just not fat and cholesterol that cause heart disease. Low fat dairy and skinless chicken even raise cholesterol. Studies have shown that chicken is as bad as red meat for raising cholesterol. Heart disease can be totally controlled by proper diet, not smoking, and exercise. Nuts and seeds are known to lower cholesterol and blood sugar levels, which lowers the risk of coronary heart disease. There are many studies that show nuts and seeds increase lifespan. Overweight individuals should be careful not to eat much more that an ounce of nuts ands seeds a day due to their high calorie content. Heart disease is completely an unavoidable disease, with the proper diet.

## Cancer.

Fruits and vegetables are correlated with longevity. Raw veggies take first place in fighting cancer. Studies on the cancer fighting abilities of vitamin C, vitamin A and folate have mixed reviews. Some studies show a slight increase and others show a slight decrease on their abilities to fight cancer. Cruciferous vegetables (kale, watercress, cauliflower, arugula, collards, and bokchoy) are the most cancer fighting foods known. Beans have additional cancer fighting abilities against reproductive cancers like breast and prostate. Studies have shown that vegetarians who eat lots of refined foods have a higher risk of cancer than a meat eater that also eats fruits and vegetables. It is suggested that if you have heart disease or family history of cancer, one should avoid eating, all meat and refined food. A study called "The China Project" came to the conclusion that people that ate vegetarian diets half their lives lived 13 years longer.

We Americans eat way to much meat and dairy protein. These are know to be associated with higher cancer rates and other illnesses. I suggest that you receive most or all of your protein from vegetable sources.

Watch out for gluten in processed food, genetically modified foods (GMOs) and added hormones in meat and dairy because they have been linked to cancer. Read labels and research what you are eating.

Early puberty is also a risk factor for cancer. High hormone levels are associated with cancer. Children that reach puberty later in life are maturing slower and live longer. People with slow metabolism have the potential to live the longest. Excess growth means that we aging quickly. Let this be a warning to weight lifters that want unnatural muscle growth by consuming vast amounts of animal proteins and even steroids. You are shortening your lives and risking cancer! Grilling, frying and barbequing meat adds even more cancer causing compounds and trans-fats, adding to the likelihood of cancer. Preventing cancer by diet and exercise has better results than mammograms and other cancer detection tests.

## The Common Cold

The common cold may negatively affect one's exercise regiment. It is possible that a cold will lead to bronchitis, croup, pneumonia, strep throat and other ailments. Washing the hands is the best way to avoid catching a cold. Rest and good nutrition are essential for recovery of a cold. One should avoid milk because it releases histamine, which causes a runny nose. Vitamin supplements are known to help if a proper diet is lacking. Vitamin A, vitamin B complex, vitamin C, zinc and copper work particularly well.

## Diabetes

This is a disease that can be control and even cured with proper exercise and diet, so it's worth talking about. It is disease where the body does not produce or use insulin. When insulin levels are low the cells of the body cannot extract glucose form the bloodstream. Glucose is a cells primary food, and a lack of glucose causes all kinds of problems, premature death being one of these. More than 80% of people with type 2 diabetes dies of a heart attacks or strokes. More than a third of all type 1 diabetics die of a heart attack before age 50. Even 10 to 20 pounds of excess weight can cause diabetes. Most diabetes patients can be cured if a good diet is practiced. 2 pounds of fresh vegetables a day with no processed, fatty, sugary, or salty food is a good diet. All diabetics should consult their physician when changing one's diet.

## The Flu

The flu is a contagious respiratory illness. It is a serous virus that cause 36,00 deaths a year. It is transmitted by sneezes or coughs being inhaled. Touching an infected surface, nasal secretions, transmitted by saliva, feces or blood can be ways to catch the Flu. The flu can remain infectious for a week. Many Flu strains can be killed by disinfectants and detergence No, one should every exercise why having the Flu.

## Obesity

Obesity is a chronic condition cause by excess body fat. Body fat is necessary for heat insulation, storing energy, organ and limb protection and other important factors. Normal body fat for men is 18%-23% in men and 25%-30% in women. Men with over 25% body fat and women over 30% body fat are considered obese. About 33% of the adult population is obese and 25% of children are obese. It is estimated that obesity will be at 50% of our population by 2030. It is a completely curable disease and 30 years ago obesity wasn't a problem. Obesity increases your risk of, coronary heart disease, diabetes, stroke, cancers, gynecological problems, hypertension, osteoarthritis, and sleep apnea, liver and gull bladder problems and so on.

Obesity can be caused by genetics, physical inactivity, frequency of eating, overeating, psychological factors and medications. Genetically, you have a much greater chance of being obese if one parent is obese. People who are sedentary burn fewer calories; so they are at greater risk of obesity. Yes people who work behind a computer screen have higher risks of disease than does a laborer. This contradicts the idea of an office job being better than a laborer. Over eating leads to weight gain. Foods high in sugar and fats exacerbate the problem. It is also know that eating large meals instead of many small meals will raise insulin levels, which in turn increases fat. One's emotional state also influences eating habits. Many find comfort in binge eating when they are sad, angry, anxious or bored. People who take antidepressants, diabetes medications, certain hormones, and anticonvulsive, are at risk for obesity. Obesity can be avoided with a good diet. You can eat all the fresh vegetables you can shove down your throat and you will never gain weight. Watch for added hormones in your meat and dairy. This has been proven to make you gain weight and cause almost every know disease.

## Osteoporosis

Osteoporosis is the reduction of bones density, causing bones to be week and fragile. It is usually caused by inadequate calcium and or vitamin D. People can be unaware of this condition until it's too late and they break a bone. The elderly are particularly at risk. Hip and spine fractures are common which lead to all kinds of other problems. Salt and sugar deplete the body of calcium. Vitamin D and calcium are required, in adequate amount, for health bones. Menopause can also cause rapid loss in bone density. Supplements should be taken if diet doesn't meet your requirements.

Total calcium intake should be less than 2000mg a day. About 1000 mg a day in needed for most men and women. Pregnant, nursing, and postmenopausal women (not on estrogen) require 1200mg to 1500mg a day.

Vitamin D requirement are 200 IU daily for men and women 19-50 years old, 400 IU for men and women 51-70 years old and 600iu for men and women over 71 years old. Weight baring exercises, like the elliptical machine and my dumbbell exercises, along with proper nutrition will help fight, if not cure osteoporosis.

## Sleep

Studies have shown that the body detoxifies during sleep and only getting 6 hours of sleep in not enough to detoxify. Lack of sleep is also correlated to many illnesses. Lack of sleep lowers your immune system and cognitive abilities. Lack of sleep creates dangerous situations. Eating well and getting exercise is the best remedy for insomnia. Sleeping on the back with a firm mattress is advised. This promotes proper breathing with the diaphragm. Sleeping on the back is also good for the posture.

## Seniors and the Importance of Nutrition with age

As the body ages, it goes through physiological changes. Whether they are caused genetically or by external factors (trauma, illness, socioeconomic conditions and so on), these changes will affect one's quality of life. Maintaining or starting a well balanced diet with a variety of foods will reduce the risk that come with aging like heart disease, diabetes, stroke and osteoporosis. Salt and sugar deplete many minerals including calcium from our bodies. It's important to include your daily requirement of Calcium, iron, fiber, protein, vitamin C, vitamin and folate. Resent studies have shown that folate taken in a supplement can cause cancer. However if folate comes from vegetables, it fights cancer. A diet low in salt, fat, and sugar is also a good suggestion. One should eat plenty of fruits and vegetables with lots of fiber. Nutrient dense or foods high in micronutrients are recommended to eliminate unnecessary calories (empty calories). Proper nutrition will slow the aging processes like muscle and bone loss, macular degeneration, Memory loss, loss of hearing, hormonal changes and painful or weakened joints. May I suggest Dr Joel Fuhrman's diet? It really is so far more advanced than any other diet with great tasting recipes as well.

Osteoporosis (low bone mass), as I mentioned before, cause bones to become week and fragile. This being cause by either a lack of vitamin D or calcium. You are required to get 400ius to 600ius per day of vitamin D and 100mg to 1500mg of calcium a day. Eliminate all unnecessary salt, sugar and fat form your diet! In a study women that drank 3-4 cups of milk a day were more likely to suffer bone fractures. Once again, say no to dairy! Don't be fooled by milk advertisements stating milk is good for osteoporosis.

Calcium loss can also be contributed to animal protein, salt, caffeine, refined sugar, alcohol, nicotine, aluminum-containing antacids, steroids, antibiotics and vitamin A supplements. Green vegetables, beans, sesame seeds, tofu and oranges are high in vitamin C without the problems that dairy has. There is lots of evidence that suggest that taking vitamin D supplements would help 3 out of 4 Americans when it comes to fracture and fall prevention.

Sarcopenia is the loss of muscle mass. As we age, we decreasingly lose the ability to regenerate new protein which leads to muscle loss We lose about 35% to 40% between the ages of 20 to 80. About 25% of our population is effected. Although, the effects of sarcopenia are not as pronounced as with osteoporosis, but it may lead to the loss of strength and mobility, which can lead to falls. 400IUs to 100IUs supplements of vitamin E can reduce the loss of muscle mass. Creatine supplement of 3-5 grams and Camosine 1000mg is also recommended to build muscle mass.

Decreased metabolic rate occurs as we age. This occurs as a direct result for loss of muscle mass. This will cause you to get fat, unless you eat less and exercise.

Arthritis is the inflammation of joints resulting from an infection, a disease, or a genetic defect. Sometimes it's inevitable as we age. 1 in 5 have signs of arthritis. Early and aggressive management of this disease will reduce complication. Glucosamine, chondroitin sulfate, and MSN are natural compounds that have great results in combating arthritis. Once again, a proper diet can eliminate this condition. Many have used fish oil to fight arthritis, and it works for many. It is now being discovered that there are some problems with fish oil. One, is that most of the oil in the capsules has turned rancid, which stresses the liver. Fish oils can also contain a wide range of PCBs and mercury. In addition, large amounts of fish oil will hinder your immune system and lower your killer T cells. Of coarse if you find that fish oil does help your condition then only take the most highly purified and free of PCBs and mercury. The active ingredient in fish oil is DHA. This can also be manufactured from algae and has none of the bad side effects as does fish oil. Many of the drugs that are used to control arthritis cause cancer.

Vision loss is a big concern as we age. 1 in 3 adults, over 65, experience some sort of vision loss. Macular degeneration, glaucoma, cataract, diabetic retinopathy, can be helped or prevented by proper nutrition. Fruits, vegetables, particularly dark leafy green veggies high in zinc, are recommended. Avoid large amount of saturated fats and sugars, because they can increase your risks. Lutein and omega-3 fatty acids (found in fish) also help.

Hearing loss is probable the most chronic conditions effecting aging adults. Over the age of 70, 90% of people suffer from hearing loss. Reducing noises, like television and music can help prevent hearing loss. Vitamins A, B, C, D, Carnitine and cysteine are important in fighting hearing loss.

Reduced mental activity is a normal part of aging. However there are many ways to combat memory loss and improve cognitive skills. As we get older, the hippocampus becomes vulnerable to deteriorations. Neurons are lost which causes our ability to process information is affected. A decrease in blood flow adds to this problem because of the lack of nutrients into the brain cells. This limits the brains ability to absorb, process, retrieve and store information. A good diet with lots of exercise is the best way to fight memory loss. Antioxidants and B vitamins (especially B-12) are important to reduce the structural loss of neurons. You should avoid a diet high in saturated fats and trans fats to keep cholesterol down and reduce the risk of stroke. Animal protein has been associated with dementia, bone loss, cancer and raised cholesterol. In fact that meat eaters (including fish and chicken) are twice as likely to get dementia.

Age related hormonal changes occur as we age. Sex hormones, estrogen and progesterone, decrease in women, Testosterone levels usually decrease in men. The pancreas will secrete higher levels of insulin and become less glucose tolerant. Making diabetes easier to develop. The urinary system, Vasopressin lowers and urine production increases. In addition the bladder loses elasticity, which contributes to nocturia (waking up to urinate).

Growth Hormone decreases as we age. This will lead to a reduction of lean body mass (muscle), which usually increases body fat.

To fight the effects of hormonal changes it is suggested that an aging adults eat 5 to 6 small meals a day to reduce blood sugar spikes and insulin levels. Maintaining a high protein diet will help support hormone secretion. Maintain a diet with enough protein to help support hormone secretion. It is important to eat small nutritious meals 4 or more time a day to ensure proper protein levels. Unless you prefer to fast like some nutritionist believe to be beneficial. Try to get your protein from vegetables or fish because to much dairy and meat protein cause cancer and other illnesses.

One needs to find humor in one's life. Life is full of tragedies and disappointments. Humor neutralizes stress. And stress kills. It's as simple as that. So don't be grump. Smile and enjoy the ride through life.

If you have questions about nutrition and exercise, videos, online consultations are available. Contact me at <u>keithnull@comcast.net</u> for info.

# ACKNOWLEDGEMENTS

1. Bruce lee and his book, "TAO of JEET KUNE DO". Thanks For the inspiration and education.
2. Joel Fuhrman, M.D., and his book, "EAT TO LIVE", Thanks for the nutrition advice and delicious recipes.
3. Gary Null, PH.D., and his books, "ULTIMATE LIFETIME HEALING" and "The Complete Encyclopedia of NATURAL HEALING". Thanks for the healing advice, nutrition and recipes.
4. "The Physiological Basis of Physical Education and Athletes". By Fox, Bowers, Foss. Thanks for the knowledge of biomechanics.
5. "Biology of Aging". By James L. Christian and John M. Gryzbowski.
6. To all the people that came to me for exercise and fitness advice. Thanks for the trust.
7. Temple University dept of Kinesiology. Thanks for the great education.
8. Sheet Metal Workers Local 19. Thanks for allowing me to pursue two very worthy careers.
9. John's Hopkins University.
10. Last but not least, Thanks to my family and friends for all the support.

www.ingramcontent.com/pod-product-compliance
Lightning Source LLC
Chambersburg PA
CBHW050406290526
45786CB00003B/1142